THE TENDER BUD

THE TENDER BUD

A Physician's Journey Through Breast Cancer

Madeleine Meldin

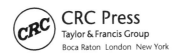

CRC Press
Taylor & Francis Group
Boca Raton London New York

CRC Press is an imprint of the
Taylor & Francis Group, an **informa** business

First published 1993 by The Analytic Press

Published 2018 by CRC Press
Taylor & Francis Group
6000 Broken Sound Parkway NW, Suite 300
Boca Raton, FL 33487-2742

Fisrt issued in paperback 2018

© 1993 by Taylor & Francis Group, LLC
CRC Press is an imprint of Taylor & Francis Group, an Informa business

No claim to original U.S. Government works

ISBN-13: 978-1-138-87246-2 (pbk)
ISBN-13: 978-0-88163-157-9 (hbk)

Visit the Taylor & Francis Web site at
http://www.taylorandfrancis.com

and the CRC Press Web site at
http://www.crcpress.com

Typeset in 11 point Goudy by Lind Graphics, Upper Saddle River, NJ

Library of Congress Cataloging-in-Publication Data

Meldin, Madeleine.
    The tender bud : a physician's journey through breast cancer /
Madeleine Meldin.
       p.   cm.
    ISBN 0-88163-157-4
    1. Meldin, Madeleine—Health.   2. Breast—Cancer—Patient—United
States—Biography.   3. Women physicians—United States—Biography.
I. Title.
    [DNLM: 1. Breast Neoplasms—diagnosis—personal narratives.
2. Breast Neoplasms—therapy—personal narratives.   3. Physicians.
Women—personal narratives.   WZ   100 M518]
RC280.B8M45   1993
362.1'9699449'092—dc20
[B]
DNLM/DLC
for Library of Congress   92-49967
                                                              CIP

For canker vice the sweetest buds doth love.
Sonnet LXX – William Shakespeare

I dedicate this book to us women on whose breasts all psychic life finds its foundation.

I dedicate it to our breasts, our maternal and womanly fountains of sustenance for children and grownups.

I dedicate it to celebrate those eternal sacred mountains, where life begins, tenderness is found, love blossoms, and myth is conceived.

I dedicate it to us women who have to surrender one or both of them to preserve our lives.

I dedicate it for us to mourn together in choral lamentation the loss of so precious an organ, so sacred a flesh.

I dedicate it for us to go on knowing that a woman's breast, even if lost to cancerous invasion, does not change the woman who has made her breast the source of love and human rest. That woman is a breast.

THE TENDER BUD

Contents

Prologue

Life is a journey we have not asked to undertake. We find ourselves on it, and most of us *expect* to complete it, to get off at the last stop, where the itinerary reaches its planned end.

Once it has become ours we feel entitled to life and to what we want to do with it. We *expect* it to continue its course, a natural cycle we observe in the fruits of the earth: the spring bud blooms, the summer fruit swells, and the fall brings to it the mellow fullness and the sweet fragrance announcing the ripeness of the completed time. Then it is the season to leave the tree of life and enter the winter rest.

Trees and fruits do not seem aware of themselves. They have the simplicity of being what they are without pretense or demand. Not so with us, self-aware creatures of the earth, conscious flesh, reflective life in process, collaborators in the fruit-making process of our own being.

We know that death may claim our lives at any time. We know it. We are certain of it. Yet we do not know it. We cannot imagine death. Our imagination, failing the task, seems to give us permission to feel immortal and entitled to our personal lives, even if others around us succumb to death each day.

The assumption about our immortality works well until our body sends some unwelcome signals that something is wrong. At that moment, we fear that death may be calling at our door to claim for itself the only life we have. Then we run to a physician to wrestle against death. The physician's words themselves have the capacity to name what ails our existential future. They may simply declare us free of the grip of death or announce a suspended or immediate death sentence. We never know what wellsprings of hope and of despair run inside us until we are confronted with the announcement of probable or impending death. The doctor's sober statement, "You have cancer," awakens within us the clamoring of a thousand voices, calling every system of defense we have to battle, to rebellion, to revolt.

We enter a dimension of reality we have not known until this moment of direct confrontation with death. Our lives turn around upon themselves, bringing into question everything we have taken for granted. Nothing is left untouched. We feel a need to explain our identity, to interrogate our past and present loves, to scrutinize the itinerary we have followed. We query, accuse, forgive, blame, pardon, pity, curse in a bewildered oscillation between fear and hope, hatred and compassion.

We physicians have joined a profession to help others in their desperate fight against untimely death. We have sworn to do everything possible to keep people alive. The medical profession's commitment, a vast enterprise of centuries of dedicated clinicians and researchers, has fulfilled its promise to eradicate human diseases that devastated large populations of the earth centuries ago, last century, or even this century: the plague, leprosy, tuberculosis, childhood infections. Hormonal, enzymatic,and genetic research has alleviated the suffering of many and managed, by very simple means, to enrich the quality of life of people who would have been crippled in the past.

These great medical achievements have had two major consequences. They have increased our feelings of *entitlement* to life, our conviction that we can *demand* that our doctors keep us alive. They have given the entire field of medicine, including medical education, a sense of power and well-deserved pride that medicine can overcome disease and human suffering. Such determination to vanquish illness is the foundation of the most astonishing achievements of modern medicine, and it deserves our gratitude and admiration. It has, however, a drawback. It places the full attention of the physician on the illness, the enemy to be conquered. I remember with fondness the battle cry of one of my doctors once when I had a bad intestinal infection. She said, raising a combative fist into the air, "We [she and I] let them [the germs] have it!" I was grateful that she had included me as a fellow fighter ready to fight with her. My illness, however, was not a deadly threat. I joined her for the sport of it.

It was another matter when Dr. Robbins said to me, as kindly as he could, "Dr. Meldin, you have an invasive carcinoma of the breast" and added a few days later, after my mastectomy, "You have metastatic axillary lymph nodes. I recommend chemotherapy to prevent the spreading of metastatic cancer." Now the sport was gone. All my doctors made a commitment to eradicate the cancer from my body. I, myself, was the battlefield and the one who could die in the middle of it. If there was to be a casualty, it could only be me.

Doctors, nurses, friends, colleagues were kind and generous with me. Only a few failed me. Kindness, however, could not reach me where I was alone with my endangered life. We are born alone; we face death alone. We have no choice. No one can do it for us.

Facing deadly illness and death does not require isolation. The patient need not be left without guidance on the internal journey of facing the terrifying threat of death. This journey is as significant as the treatment itself. If the body is cured but fear of death overtakes the mind of the survivor, the restored life may lose its zest, its joy. For a person to be fully restored, the physician must have conquered the illness, and the patient must have accepted the challenge of mortality.

Doctors are not trained to study and attend to the psychic process elicited by illness. The patient's unavoidable psychic suffering follows certain patterns and paths that can be mapped out to offer some guidance. The confrontations, the fear, the shame, the bewildering fantasies, the humiliating wishes for protection, the retreat from physical and emotional pain are unavoidable experiences encountered by all patients. The most painful feeling of all is the unnecessary conviction that such suffering can neither be revealed nor be made part of the process of being ill itself. The pain of such isolation can and must be alleviated.

Being a physician, as I am, does not assuage the existential pain of the threat of death. As clinicians in charge, we are used to facing the death of *others*. As the professional masters of life-defending techniques, we find in the experience of our own frightened and bewildered response to a deadly illness a source of shame and humiliation, a paradoxical reaction to the human impotence that death imposes on us.

Death strips us of all titles and decorations. It leaves us facing our common human fragility. A deathly ill physician is simply a person in medical and existential crisis in need of competent colleagues and compassionate friends. Until health returns, the physician can only speak with a patient's voice. Someone must hear the cries and whispers, and respond.

In other encounters with the unknown, we avail ourselves of guides, whether commercial or spiritual. To travel we have travel agents; to learn we have teachers; to address transcendent realities we have ministers, priests, rabbis. Why should it be that to travel the desert of the fear of death we should walk without a companion? There is no need. Others have traveled it. Some have lived; some have died. Those who have returned from the valley of death can guide their fellow pilgrims so that they will not be so afraid of being afraid. They can show physicians, nurses, health care professionals, relatives, and friends the landmarks, the pitfalls, the turning points of fear and hope in a journey of dark and ominous suffering.

In this book I have written of my own experience as a cancer patient. I did not write it initially for publication. I have always suspected autobiographical indulgence. I wrote it out of need, because I was a patient trembling in dark uncertainty. It has not been editorially embellished; the only editorial corrections were for grammar, style, and syntax. This is, therefore, a document, the narrative of an ordinary patient who happens to be a physician, describing the vicissitudes of her personal life during her breast cancer diagnosis and treatment. The dates in each of the chapters signify the days when I made the entries in my journal. I wrote as soon as I could after the events transpired. I was teaching a new course, seeing my patients, and trying to behave normally. I could not write every day or even every week. Sometimes I had to wait for several weeks before I could write about what I was feeling.

The impetus to make my journal public came from colleagues and my own doctors, who, knowing what I was writing, wanted to read what I was saying to myself. When I had enough distance from my experience, I gave them my manuscript. They all felt that I should publish it, that it would be of help to other patients and to all that care for them. I accepted their suggestion in my wish to offer my own experience to other women and men who feel alone upon hearing the fateful phrase: "You have cancer."

I hope that reading about the sorrows and hopes of my journey offers them some point of comparison to understand their own suffering.

1

Discovery

December 29

All was now ready: tickets, phone calls, office care. One more month and winter in the U.S.A. would become summer in the Caribbean. The alarm sounded at 6:00 A.M. as it had done for the last 40 years since I was a girl of 13. I got up and said my "Our Father" to join the sun and all creation, human and beast, angel and virus, in the entrance into this new day as inaugural as any other day since the beginning of time.

I pushed on the TV button to catch the news left behind as I slept while (unlike myself as a girl of 13 who got up at six) I made my bed, feeling virtuous and self-contented. There was no news today. There was only the usual: the bickering in Washington, the war between Iran and Iraq, and the oppression of blacks in South Africa. Enough. The atomic bombs had not left the silos. Men in government were crazy in their normal ways. I could begin the day and take care of my present without the interference of history-making history. I went down to the office, put on the heater and the humidifier, closed the door to the study, checked that everything was in place in the office and in the waiting room, and finally unlocked the door for the first patient to come in. Then I went to the kitchen. The sun was still below the horizon, but the clearing sky announced its coming. The kettle had enough water for a cup of tea. It would boil while I showered. Then the tea could brew in the hot cup while I did my aerobic exercises.

I started the shower to get it warm and pushed the button to hear more news from the public radio station. The news continued to be banal and warming. There were some stories about dinosaur bones in Colorado and a woman 105 years old in Alabama.

The hot water warmed me too. I thought about the joy and good luck of us Americans and citizens of Western civilization who get such a wonderful rain of hot water on ourselves just by turning a knob. All the while we take it so for granted. On the radio I heard the voice of a homeless person living in a cardboard home in Los Angeles: "The shade is better than the open air, but it has no facilities like a hotel – no bathroom, no showers." I felt grateful and inhaled the warm vapor while delighting in the lilac scent of the soap.

Then, there under the soft lustrous skin, the finger felt something, something I did not want my finger to feel. But it did feel it – a small, slightly elongated hard mass in the right breast. A barrage of denying thoughts fired from my brain, like a well-trained team of artillery men firing in orderly succession. Boom! "That is not a node." Boom! "It is only the progesterone you are taking." Boom! "It is just the mammary tissue." Boom! "It is not really hard." Boom! "It can be a cyst." Boom! "Don't exaggerate. That is nothing." Boom! "Quit examining." Boom! "There is no cancer in our family." Boom! "Don't make it cancer." Boom! "If you keep on touching it, you'll make it bigger." Boom. . . .

Slowly I began to emerge from the shooting of the artillery. The medical fingers became professional. They examined, noticed, recognized, explored the neighboring areas. Then I said, "You have a small node in your right breast. The consistency is cystic. Wait a couple of days. Examine it carefully. If it is still there, then get an examination at once."

My brain began a new type of firing. Now it functioned like a computer, accumulating one-line sentences against the until-now unthinkable thought: breast cancer.

"Your mammogram was normal."
"Dr. Barron's office did not call you."
"There is not one case of breast cancer in your family."
"You have been taking estrogen and progesterone as prescribed for breast cancer prevention."

"Your adipose tissue index is low."
"You have never smoked."
"You eat healthful food."
"You exercise every day."

I had the feeling that I was appealing my case in front of a tribunal that was about to pass a final judgment. I wanted to convince them that *I* should not have cancer, least of all breast cancer. I felt aware that I was being persuasive in making my case, bringing in factors that would make it impossible to conclude that *I* had cancer.

Working was a very hard task. My mind had no other interest but to argue my case. I decided to work in battle with myself, to listen to my patients, to feel their feelings, to understand what they also were afraid to understand. I earned my bread with the sweat of my brow.

Trying to distract myself proved arduous. When the work day was over, my mind perched successively on the shoulders of every one of my critics in the past and its furious firing began again.

Boom! "You are making a mountain out of a molehill." Boom! "What are you complaining about? That is nothing" Boom! "You are *always* so certain. You get all excited and imagine things." Boom! "Forget it, You are always bothering people with your little complaints. All that noise for a puffed rice size little lump." Boom! "The doctor will laugh when you, a doctor, arrive in a panic with such a lousy little thing. Forget it!" Boom! "Stop thinking. Anyone would think you are dying of cancer. You exaggerate. You *always* exaggerate."

I stopped myself after having fallen flat on my face, hit by so many critics. I got up slowly to recover my dignity. I told myself, "Cancer is nothing to play around with. It is a subtle and terrible enemy. I shall do what I promised. If tomorrow it is there, I shall call the doctor the day after and have it all carefully checked."

I dreamed of a storm and floods in a valley with nearby mountains I had seen on a trip to Machu Pichu. I woke up and thought of some Peruvian hills called by the local people *Nono*. They have that name because they are shaped like two breasts, and *Nono*, the guide told us, is the Quechua name for breasts.

I repeated the routine of the previous day as though life were following its natural path, while I, for the first time was afraid of my body, of showering, of finding that small grain of puffed rice at the tip of my right breast. I needed willpower to bring my medical fingers to the right upper tip of my right breast. *It was there.* It was slightly bigger, hard, and firm to palpation. The surrounding tissues were normal. "Tomorrow I shall call the doctor," I resolved. I could not do it today. All of me – mind, body, soul, I, my past, my future – did not want to hear today that I had breast cancer.

My mind took over again. This time I envisioned the grotesque parade of the dead. Elizabeth, my girlhood friend of 41 years, was the first one to appear, looking corpselike as she had the last time we talked together so tenderly, so sadly, so painfully. Her last wish was, "Please take me to see the lake. I want to smell the air, to see the mountains and the water." We had to carry her there bodily. There were others in the parade, the ones I knew personally and the ones whose stories I had heard about. I felt fear, the cold fear of a prolonged death. Images of nursing homes in New York City returned like apocalyptic visions, showing in front of me white bones rising from beds of sorrow.

The morning weather was gray and gloomy; so was I. Integrity and will power brought me back to my work, and it was a blessing to work. I felt grateful to my patients. I wanted to thank them for telling me their thoughts and feelings. Listening to them was healing the premonition of death in me. They were alive, wrestling with life and with me. I felt particularly grateful to those who wanted to fight with me or who complained about me. It was an indicator – unknown to them – that they considered me a living and strong enemy for today's battle. In my heart I thanked them for making me participate in the fight of life. I was also grateful that they would continue to come, not abandoning me to this inner enemy installed in my breast. I had a wish to say something soft, compassionate, kind, to each of them. Perhaps I wanted to soothe myself in them. I did not. I supervised my every word, my every thought. I had to remain *their* doctor, regardless of what I felt. I had to attend to *their* pain, whether or not I had my own. A feeling of dignified pride sustained my self-monitoring task. At the end of the day I felt like a laborer who has faithfully carried her bricks to the point of construction. And I felt exhausted, lonely, and alone with this unshareable secret. I had to talk to my doctor. I could no longer be alone with this knowledge. Nobody else, not even my best friends, could say anything until a medical examination had been performed on my breast.

My gynecologist, a very good man, had retired six months earlier. He had referred his patients to two doctors, and I had selected Dr. Marcus, a woman, and had my records sent to her. Now was the time to make her acquaintance. I called the office. The secretary, said with a condescending tone, that Dr. Marcus did not have time for at least five weeks. I said, "I am 53 years old, and I have a lump in my breast. I must see her immediately." She argued that it was impossible. She could send me to another doctor. I retorted that Dr. Marcus had all my records and previous mammograms. I had to be seen by her at once. The secretary claimed that it was impossible. I requested that she inform the doctor immediately about my demand to be seen at once because of my age and the nature of my node. Then, miraculously, she found an hour four days later. I had won a battle of wills, a life-saving battle of wills that I should not have had to fight. I imagined the shy and frightened clerks and housewives, incapable of fighting a dictatorial secretary who governs the doctor's schedule like an old fashioned courtier closing off access to the queen. I imagined their cancers growing, invading the lymph nodes and bones, and the secretary polishing her fingernails while answering their anguished phone calls. I am not in favor of lawsuits, but there is something terribly irresponsible and uncaring about a secretary who deals with matters of life and death as though she were dispensing favors by virtue of *her* power to control access to the doctor.

The doctor, a woman in her late 30s, was pleasant, well mannered, and obviously knowledgeable. She had read my record and knew my medical history. She established the rules of our relationship in a polite manner. She proceeded to examine me. Her fingers explored my breast with precise tactile questioning, knowingly stopping where the underlying surface indicated pathology. She found the node and informed me that it seemed like a cyst. Hopefully, I agreed. Under the pressure of my own fingers, the node had the tense, elastic consistency of a tightly contained liquid mass. She informed me that she was going to aspirate the liquid or whatever else she would find. Her surgical technique left nothing to be desired; it was gentle, unhesitant, efficient. She sighed joyously, "I have good news for you. It is a cyst. The liquid is milky, a bit cloudy, with some fat particles. It seems like a typical cyst. However, to cover every possibility I am sending it to the pathologist. I'll be surprised if it's worse than a cyst."

I asked to see the liquid. It looked a little like diluted milk, with

small whitish particles and slightly larger fat grains, a perfectly innocent and esthetically pleasant liquid. I felt a certain warm feeling of
gratitude toward it. Its benign appearance seemed to cleanse me of my
images of dreadful cancerous cells invading my breast.

I dressed while chatting with the doctor about these kinds of
milk-duct cysts and their benign prognosis. I informed her that I had
a trip abroad scheduled a month hence. She said the report should be
in in a week.

I wanted to believe what I had seen: a cystic liquid, mischievously
frightening me with the unthinkable word "cancer." But I did notice
something. I was afraid to fully inform myself about what I had
noticed: the node did not disappear after the aspiration. I knew what
that meant: either there was more liquid there in another cystic
compartment (an unlikely hope), or there was a solid mass of tissue, of
cancerous tissue. I chose to believe it was a cyst. My option was
incomplete. I called Joe, an experienced gynecologist and very close
friend. He asked me to describe it all carefully. I did. "Don't you
worry," he said. "Everything you say points in the direction of a cyst."

My wish to believe that it was only a cyst gained the upper hand,
and I declared myself free of cancer. I had a good reason. This was an
important moment in my life. In six days I was to deliver a very
important lecture, the culmination of some research I had been
carrying out for years. I was proud to be asked to present my work to
a group of reputable scholars. I had polished my presentation to its
finest details. Gregory and Carmen, a couple of academicians and very
close friends, helped with editing and my style of delivery. A moment
of intellectual glory was coming, and I was determined to enjoy it fully.

The lecture went very well. The room was packed and the audience
attentive. The question-and-answer period was an enjoyable exercise
in intellectual agility. I savored the moment and the dinner that
followed. The following day I consulted some colleagues, and we
agreed on the journal to which to submit my presentation for publication. I decided to call the editor, who most graciously agreed to
review it. "Now," I said to myself, "is the time to start getting ready to
teach a course next semester at the university, and I should keep
writing about this subject that has brought me a pinch of academic
glory."

Life was rolling along full of satisfactions crowned with a serene
feeling of accomplishment. The following morning's mail brought the

usual mixture of junk mail, personal messages, and a letter from the gynecologist. It was brief: "Dear Doctor Meldin: Please contact me immediately for further care of your condition." Signed, Dr. Marcus. The severity of the language foretold ominous news, or, to say it simply, the only news that it could be–cancer.

I called at once. Her account of the pathologist's report contained the euphemism a doctor uses to modulate the patient's fear of the worst. "The pathologist does not like the alignment of some cells in the sample I sent him. He suggests a biopsy to clarify the diagnosis. He cannot write a report with the information at hand." Fear did not cloud my judgment. "I want to have a biopsy immediately," I said.

"You know that time is of the essence," the doctor said. She promised to get an appointment with a surgeon as soon as possible. I was free that afternoon. Two hours later I was talking with the surgeon. The biopsy was arranged for six days later. I knew that my chances of having cancer were now very, very high. Fear, horror, and disbelief intermingled as I beheld the procession of cancerous women I have known–the living and the dead– those crippled by the experience of the treatment, those capable of standing tall in the face of tragedy even to the end. It did not matter much if they were crippled or standing tall. I was always moved to great pity by their suffering, their ruined bodies, their concentration camp looks during the period of chemotherapy. Now, *they*, from whom I distanced myself by the powerful subtlety of the pronoun "they," were getting very close to me, stretching out their bald heads and maimed chests to show me that I too could be one of them, one of those cancerous people who incarnate in their signs and wounds the faded tuberculous and lepromatous faces of the past. These are the forbidden faces of human doom.

Waiting, like waiting for Godot, is a long, despairing, lonely act, nervously filled with ceaseless looking in all directions, expecting it, it, just *it*, just it to come, to come forth.

The days of waiting ended on that Tuesday, exactly six days from the moment I had heard the medical euphemism about "cells aligned in a way the pathologist does not like." That morning, as if all were normal, I saw three patients, from 7:00 to 9:40, as though my questions and carefully worded utterances to my patients could, in fact, undo the pathogenic power of a harmful "alignment of thoughts and feelings" in their minds and lives. The parallel construction of hopeful wishing made my work an act of displaced magic on my own behalf.

At 10:30 I was on the other side of the patient–doctor relationship. A bracelet was put on me to identify my body. I was given a unisex gown with a print of little blue flowers on a white background. We all—men and women—looked alike in the Day Surgery Waiting Room. Our feet were dressed in foam rubber green and blue gnome like slippers, and our bodies were covered with some piece of clothing called, with charitable exaggeration, a robe.

Each of us put on a faint smile and withdrew into a private universe of fear, encircled by the armrests of our chairs. Surgeons and nurses looked like inmates of a gigantically funny nut house, with their enormous, blue-clothed shoes and their pointed hats at the two extremes of bodies, covered by blue or green operating room gowns or pants.

Every so often a nurse came to fetch one of us. The arrow was unidirectional—a one-way street—from the chair, to the stretcher, to the operating table. Soft-voiced and kind, the nurses picked us up delicately, as you pick wild flowers knowing that they are going to wither in a minute. Like a small flower left in the climber's path, I was the last one, to be picked up in my inexorable journey to the withering process. Gentle hands of maternal women helped me from table to table. In loud voices they checked my name and the nature of the procedure: right breast biopsy. Then surgeon and nurses spoke to me with the modulated tones we use when we know that terrible news must be delivered to an innocent person. As they proceeded, they grew more silent, as though the inhibition of their voices could hide from me what their eyes were seeing: a highly suspicious breast node. The surgeon, Dr. Robbins, in between caring words about whether or not it hurt, said to himself, "I am going to take another little piece in here." The medical man in him was talking to the surgeon in charge of my life, who was removing, I knew it now, as much of the cancer as possible. Then he began to close the wound. His tone was lighter. I asked about stitches. He laughed quietly, sympathetically, with me. "Only one little stitch, Dr. Meldin, one more, and then you'll be all done, and I will go down to the pathologist and come back to talk with you." I knew that he knew that I knew I had cancer, but we both respected the rules of confirmation of final factual evidence, that pretty, instantly colored slide that shows in a delicately printed pattern the cancerous cells disturbing the natural symmetry of normal tissue.

They brought me to the recovery room, where I joined the withered creatures who were trying to perk themselves up with juice and crackers. I had a few minutes to prepare myself to face what I knew Dr. Robbins was going to say. A storm of hope and fear raged in me. I imagined, against the already existing evidence, that he came in, all smiles, and said cheerfully, "You are a lucky woman, Dr. Meldin. It is only a cyst." The fear made me fear to hope. The fear raged with the words, "You do have cancer, you do, you do." It was no easy task to drink juice and munch crackers while I was a leaf in the storm of my feelings.

Suddenly he came, light footed and sober. He squatted so that his face was on a level with mine. That bodily gesture, that extra gentleness of leveling with me, had already said what he went on to say: "I am afraid that the news is bad. You do have an infiltrating carcinoma. You'll need surgery and then perhaps radiation or chemotherapy." He clarified that he might only need to take a sector of one breast, something barely noticeable. All would depend on the final report about the type of cells, their characteristics, their responsiveness to antihormones, and other factors. He was factual, respectful in his words, and compassionate in the subtleties of his face, his hands, his tone of voice.

I, the person in command of me, emerged from the chaos of feelings and said, "Dr. Robbins, you just changed my life." Then I felt I was doing him an injustice. It was *my* cancer. He had not given it to me. I said, "I am sorry. You haven't done anything. The cancer has changed my life." Having acknowledged to myself and to him that I had accepted entering the dark tunnel of CANCER, the tropical land of uncontrollable growth, I prepared myself for the uneven combat. "Dr. Robbins," I said, "I want to do anything you and I can do, promptly, efficiently, effectively. I want to have a second opinion, a second pathologist, an oncologist."

He agreed and said that it was the best course to follow. I thought of a close friend of one of my close friends, an eminent clinical oncologist. I was so shaken, so frightened that I could not remember her last name. I said her first name. Dr. Robbins smiled and found pleasure in filling in my gap with her last name. "I have some patients of hers." he said. "I know her." I wanted protection, someone, somebody to help me in this terrible encounter with cancer.

I begged, "Would you be willing to call her yourself first? Later I will call her." He agreed at once, insisting that he would facilitate whatever I wanted to do. He also clarified that he would be glad to be my surgeon but that I was free to choose another. He was at my service. I told him that I was scheduled to take a trip abroad on the 22nd of the month. Today was the ninth. I would like to have the surgery performed on the 22nd to avoid adding to my burdens that of informing my patients that I was ill—at least for the time being. He said that there was no problem scheduling it for that date and that I had a few days to inform him if that was what I wanted. He asked me if I had any other questions or requests. I had none, except a tremendous wish to be protected, saved, taken out of this nightmare, removed from the conveyor belt that circles around CANCER. I said, "Thank you. You have said as much as I need to know now. Let's proceed as fast as we can, and let's keep in touch." He shook my hand, and we formed a war pact against the infiltrator of my breast.

The nurse helped me get dressed and gave me a prescription for Darvocet in case I had pain. Once dressed, I looked exactly like the Dr. Meldin I was used to being. I recognized myself in the mirror of the dressing room. I did not feel weak. I was in full command of my 5'4" body and had all my wits about me to negotiate the labyrinthine corridors of the hospital, go out, buy my pills for minor aches, get my car from the garage, and go home.

2

The Sacrifice of the
Part for the Whole

January 4

I felt I like a Russian doll, a doll inside another doll. The outer me was my usual me, a decisive person, moved by self-determination. The doll inside me was cancerous, rendering me incompetent to control my own destiny after having taken possession of me from the inside of my unsuspecting breast. A wish to surrender emerged within me, to let the inner doll penetrate the surface of the exterior doll until she was taken over and progressively anesthetized into the sleep of death. The wish grew in proportion to the increasing awareness of the nature of the fight I was being called upon to make to stop the cancerous invasion of my body: the surrendering of my breast and the massive intake of poison to kill the cancerous doll within the surface of my skin. I felt a tremendous fatigue, beyond tears, beyond words, beyond despair, the fatigue of those who have entered the war for survival. I knew it was a war without truce until death itself came from natural causes, or other causes, or until this very same cancer caused my body to add a minuscule pile of dust to the universal ground.

I arrived home dazed, shrouded in the cloud formed by the echoing words, "You have an infiltrating carcinoma." I called the friend who was a friend of the woman oncologist and left a message on his machine. "Alexander, please call me back as soon as possible. I have disturbing news about myself." I sat down, trying to think, to feel, to be. I had to think carefully and clearly about what to do, whom to call first, how to go about consulting truly knowledgeable people, and how to do it in a very short time in order to cram everything into my "vacation" to the Caribbean.

Alexander called back, his voice indicating that he understood that something grave had happened. I told him as simply as I could, "Alexander, I have breast cancer." It saddened me to hear his shock and despair. I knew that it pained him to hear that I was a cancer victim. I felt the fear of having to deliver the news to many other friends, bringing to them the sadness and grief I had just brought to Alexander. I needed them, their help, their support, their compassion, their sorrow, their fear. I harbored a secret wish that Alexander could do something marvelous, miraculous, to make it all go away. Maybe he knew a doctor who could make it vanish, some magic new enzyme, some laser beam, something, anything. While I was going through this inner frenzy, Alexander was talking about contacting Sara, a reputable oncologist, and about how she could help me select some top consultants. At his suggestion I called her at once. I knew her socially through him. I knew her parents, her husband and her children. They were a good family with whom I had shared many delightful moments.

Sara called back at once. She reacted as Alexander had, indicating by her words and tone of voice the sorrow she felt about my having breast cancer. I knew then, in my second call, that I was going to assume the task of messenger of bad news—a "*kakos angelos,* an angel of bad news," I said to myself, playing with the Greek words. She said she knew exactly the best physicians for me to consult and asked me whether I was willing to accept any time they had available to see me. I said that I was. This was a top priority for me. If I had to reschedule patients, I had to reschedule patients. She promised to get back to me the following day. She did. Dr. Nagle, the oncologist, was to see me on Monday at 10:00 AM and Dr. Hughes, the radiologist, on Tuesday at 10:00 AM. Now I had to start juggling my patients' schedules. For the first time I realized that from now on I had to live with the possibility of my own unpredictability for my own patients. But what had to be done, had to be done. I sat down to see how I could accommodate all the patients without totally disturbing their lives. I could not. I had to cancel some regular patients and a consultation and reschedule a few to the evening. They all complied and seemed eager not to know the reasons for the changes.

The next 10 days were to be a frenetic race against the clock. Each day I went to the hospital three times, in between patients, measuring the seconds, carrying lunch or some snack in my pocketbook. I repeated to everyone the same litany: "I am sorry. I have limited time. I have to be back to see my own patients at such and such a time." They were all respectful, kind, and efficient. I assume that in spite of my dignified manner and professional stance they could read the anguish and fear on my face. After all, they too had learned the sober and tactful manners of messengers of bad news, as they frequently are. The personnel in oncology and radiation therapy seemed to know that we all were in death row, and they treated us with sober, honest respect. I felt an immense gratitude for all their little gestures of human kindness and for the self-contained manner by which they expressed concern. It made me feel held, cared for, without losing my dignity and my own sobriety. I was tense and charged, like an electrified wire. Any minor provocation would have gone beyond the limits of my tolerance. I knew it, and I was grateful for their respectful tact.

January 5

On Monday I met with Dr. Nagle, the first person with whom I was to talk about the simple and undeniable fact that I was now a cancer patient.

Dr. Nagle met me in a small, surgically clean examination room. He shook hands with me and tried to make me feel at ease with him. He was a mild-mannered, pleasant-looking man, obviously younger than I. He spoke softly, with a warm, ironic style capable of conveying human respect and compassion while still acknowledging the factual presence of a deadly threat.

He did not assume the superior position of one who knew what to do with me and to me. He acknowledged that before I had been a psychiatrist I had been a general practitioner for a time and that I too had been a deliverer of bad news, a *kakos angelos*. We were able to laugh with ironic sadness at the nature of our jobs: "Well, Mr. R, I have the pleasure to inform you that you have leukemia." We both knew that laughing about the truth was my way of keeping the dignified distance I needed to be able to collaborate with him, to accept my cancer and make it real and bearable.

While we talked casually like two old friends reminiscing about my past as a general practitioner, his hands explored my body, interrogating its surface softly for further hidden signs of disease. The fingers questioned each inch of my breasts and lingered seriously, reflectively, ponderously on each small indication of danger. Relieved by their inability to find another mass, they travelled to my collar bone and axilla, searching for those persisting grains of sure death, infiltrated lymph nodes. The arduous labor of the fingers had silenced the man. I missed his voice as though he had not spoken for hours. His silence filled me to the brim with fear. The unpronounceable word formed an immense sign, neonlike, blinking *on* by the switch of fear and *off* by the switch of denial. It read METASTASIS.

Finally he spoke. "The lymph nodes do not appear obviously enlarged, except as a result of the biopsy. However, as you know, there is no guarantee. Only the pathology report will tell the facts."

I got dressed, and he sat down to write his notes and discuss my options. There were but two, if the report of the pathologist indicated that option number one was even possible. Option number one was a lumpectomy (a medical neologism that is a hybrid combination of English and Greek). A sector of the breast would be removed, followed by extensive radiation. I was to discuss that option with the radiologist. Option two was mastectomy, which would or would not be followed by chemotherapy, depending on the presence or absence of lymph nodes.

I voiced my fears about my very sensitive skin and the possible complications of radiation. Much to my horror, Dr. Nagle mentioned that a woman had had a pemphigoid reaction with large blisters of the skin. As a child I had had most distressing episodes of pemphigoid urticaria, and I envisioned my skin bursting in dripping blisters. I felt fear, a wish to recoil and hide.

Then we talked about mastectomy and its advantages. The irony seemed truly excessive. In tears, I laughed, "The amazons liked it and did it for fun. I don't like it. I am not an amazon." I saw my childhood chest, showing its ribs on my right side, and I felt that half a woman was going out of me. I called myself to myself while I cried and said to Dr. Nagle, but mostly to myself, "I am a woman. I'll remain a woman.

I *am* a woman." While I spoke, the tears I was crying were shed by *me*, the me who knew I did not want to part from my breast no matter what I said. Dr. Nagle remained respectfully silent while I was crying and talking.

After a while he said, "You don't have to make any decisions now. Consult the radiation therapist tomorrow, while I wait for the pathologist's report. I'll call you at home as soon as I have it. Dr. Robbins will call you too. Then you, Dr. Robbins, Dr. Hughes, and I should make a decision."

I left in a daze. It was the 9th of December. On the 22nd I was scheduled to take a plane to the Caribbean. Instead, I was, I knew now, to take another trip, probably to the operating room to surrender my right breast. Two words began a frenetic dance in my head, faster and faster and faster, like a couple intoxicated with love or drugs: CANCER-METASTASIS . . . CANCER-METASTASIS.

I composed myself, got the car out of the garage, and drove home, having only 10 minutes left to have lunch and get ready to be on the other side of the patient–doctor relationship, to be the doctor in charge of a pained person's mind.

The following day I met with Dr. Hughes, an expert in cancer and radiation therapy and head of the hospital's breast cancer unit. I had to cancel two patients. One of them, a woman I was seeing in an extended consultation, whose previous visit I had also canceled to see Dr. Nagle, became indignant with my sloppy and unreliable manners and found herself another therapist. It was a pity because her chronic and self-defeating condition most surely required psychoanalytic psychotherapy. I knew the psychiatrist that replaced me, and I was sure he would give her some medication without psychotherapy. That young and troubled woman was the first person to pay a price for my having cancer.

I arrived at the hospital at the scheduled time. The first shock was that the receptionist happened to be an old acquaintance of mine, a lonely and empty woman who had become a professional psychosomatic patient, going from one colleague of mine to another and keeping herself busy by learning what was to be known about her therapists and their patients and then providing free gossip services to whoever wanted to know anything about anybody. It was too late to avoid her when I recognized her. I had already said the words "radiation therapy." I could see her lighting up, ready for some bad news about me. I felt anger and despair. It was not enough that I had cancer; I now had to start playing hide-and-seek, measuring my words, and acting "cool" to protect my privacy and my patients. It would be devastating to most of them to hear that I had cancer. In that instant, facing the receptionist's broad and interrogating eyes, I discovered that I had begun the career as keeper of my deadly secret. Cancer is, and must remain for a practicing psychiatrist, classified information. If one is about to die, ethics and honesty require that one protect the patients' welfare first. Then one must decide how to tell each of them individually. I was not about to die. This was a manageable illness for the time being. It would have to be yet another of the things my patients did not know about me.

Crestfallen and worried, I arrived at Dr. Hughes's office. A blonde and cheerful nurse, who called me by my first name, led me into the consulting room. Offhandedly, she asked me what town I was from and what my specialty was. I felt intruded upon, violated, even when I understood that she meant well. The offense was that she did not address *me*, the person who was here, who had left her own patients, moved by the compelling need to deal with the death she had just found installed in her own breast.

Dr. Becker, a woman resident, arrived, introduced herself, and informed me that she was taking my history on behalf of Dr. Hughes. She had arrived half an hour later than the scheduled time. I informed her that I had allotted two hours for the consultation and that I had to be back at exactly 12:25 to see a patient. We still had one hour and twenty minutes.

Dr. Becker seemed intimidated by me. She took a history in an unsystematic manner and then looked at the mammograms, confirming that they were unusual. My cancer was located exactly outside the area captured by the film. I looked at them with her, pondering details of the mammary tissue registered in the film, in particular the way in which the hormones I had been taking had kept my breasts "younger" than they actually were. Several years earlier I had a hysterectomy and had since been taking the doses of estrogen and progesterone recommended by the American Cancer Society to protect a woman from breast cancer and osteoporosis after such surgery.

Dr. Becker and I chatted about inconsequential things. The time was going by. It was close to noon, and I had only a half an hour left to decide my future with the help of Dr. Hughes. He finally came and, following the usual style of relaxing the patient, he began to talk about my specialty. I wanted to talk about myself, about the treatment, about every technical detail that could help me decide what course to follow.

I informed him of my skin problem as a possible contraindication to radiation therapy. He obviously had not read my clinical history sent by Dr. Nagle and did not know I had had pemphigoid urticaria as a child or that I had suffered from contact dermatitis. He assumed I was talking about fair skin and told me he had treated 1,000 patients, many with very fair skin, and none had had any adverse reaction. I felt angry. I did not want to be a statistic. I had already many times been part of the 1% of cases that *do not* affect the statistics but who bear the pain of the adverse consequences. I felt fear, the fear of being pushed through a conveyor belt without anybody checking what was happening to me. He kept talking: I had to go for six weeks, Monday through Friday, one hour a day, to receive the treatment. They could accommodate my schedule. I would feel very tired, because radiation is toxic to the body. While he was talking about radiation – not about my being irradiated – I kept on hearing Dr. Nagle's words, "Cells have memory. They never forget the radiation they have already received." I well understood what he meant. As a young woman of 20 I had received radiation therapy to my armpits for an intractable exudative eczema, and it was not unthinkable that the lead protection placed on my breast had not properly covered the very edge of the breast where the cancer had grown.

I had many questions to ask, but it was 12:10 and my patient was waiting for me. I told Dr. Hughes I had to go. He said I could return to talk some more. My only wish was never to need his treatment. I felt afraid to the point of terror. I felt a victim of his real science fiction gun of invisible rays directed at me, regardless of who I was or what kind of idiosyncrasies or life history I had. Bullets and weapons do not discriminate among whom they kill. They are satisfied with killing. My fantasy saw me in a Kafkaesque radiation chamber of silent, penetrating rays that attacked me while my breast wound and armpit were transforming themselves on a blistered land of scorched skin.

My decision was in the making. Unless the entire team suggested that radiation therapy was the only choice, I was going to refuse it. I did not hide the reason from myself. Radiation is really only a blind tool. Its use is based on statistics and cannot take into account the individual characteristics of the patient. It has no margins. It is only yes or no. *Me,* that poor me who so desperately needed attention, tenderness, respect, care, seemed to be best ignored by this modality of treatment. Dr. Hughes, kind and concerned as he appeared, seemed to have been shaped by the power of his tool. He too acted indiscriminately, presenting weapons and statistics to *me,* a person so frightened, so dominated, so concerned by the need to act promptly against the invasive (another warlike word) penetration of my cancer into the heart of *me.* A dark cloud enshrouded me in a mood of gloom and impotence. There was nothing else to do until Monday or Tuesday, when the pathologist would release his report and send the slides to Dr. Nagle, who would review them and show them to another pathologist. Dr. Nagle wanted to form his own, independent opinion in contemplating the best course of treatment based on the type of cells, their immaturity, their invasiveness, their potential for metastasis and their receptivity to antiestrogenic medication. His decision would also depend on whether or not the cancerous cells had hormonal receptor sites, a determination requiring a test that could be performed only a few days later.

I tried to plow ahead and do everything I had to do to go to the hospital and put my life, personal and professional, in order before I went in for surgery. So many decisions awaited me! Whom would I tell that I had cancer? Should I inform my distant relatives and my friends here and abroad? Did I have to tell my colleagues at the university and the institutions I belonged to? Would I need a nurse after the operation? How could I make the best decisions for myself? What kinds of questions did I have to ask of myself, of the surgeon, of the plastic surgeon (a character who had not as yet entered the play but whose coming was announced by Dr. Robbins)? To start, I decided to call my gynecologist and my internist to inform them about the results of the biopsy.

I first called Dr. Marcus, the gynecologist I had seen. She seemed shocked by the news that I had cancer and began to talk to me from some unknown place inside herself about coming to surgery with me and helping me out with topical hormones "when you resume normal sexual relations." We had never talked about sexual relations, and they seemed to me quite unrelated to my telling her about breast cancer. I do not know what prompted her to say "resume" as though I had stopped something that I had to restart. I was patient. I was very quickly becoming acquainted with the discomfort of my colleagues who were facing the fact that I, a member of the healing profession, was in the grips of a deadly threat. I decided to be compassionate with Dr. Marcus. Being about 18 years younger than I, with children and a husband, she was obviously feeling the horror of my cancer as though it were hers. Besides, Dr. Marcus knew that I lived alone. Her confused and confusing words could well have reflected her efforts to put herself in my shoes, while she as my doctor could do nothing to help me out as a sister in pain. I thanked her, and we both agreed to keep in touch. I never heard from her, and I learned from Dr. Robbins, to whom she had referred me, that she had never contacted him either. But even though I felt intense anger,I was beyond it, then as now. The sorrow and the fear, the acute awareness of our animal fragility and of the tragic sense of our knowing our destiny, that all-too-human knowledge of death, provided me with compassion for a young colleague who seemed to feel as pressured as I felt myself. (I had known the reluctance of delivering bad news when I was a general practitioner and had to say, "Mr. X, your cells indicate that you have an acute leukemia," knowing the patient would be dead in nine months.)

That evening my friend Alexander came to visit with two gifts, a pretty Indian silk purse that his wife, Martha, had bought in her trip to Bombay a few weeks before. It was supposed to be my birthday gift. It now became a consolation gift of sorts. Alexander also brought Rabbi Kushner's book *When Bad Things Happen to Good People*. It was their way of saying that I was a good person and that I should not have cancer. The tender and generous affection of Alexander and his family touched me with the warmth of feeling held, appreciated, attended to as me, myself, beyond cancer and death. And it felt good.

They were joined by all my shocked friends, who seemed to have agreed tacitly that I should not have cancer. Each friend tried to help in the way she or he could. Rachel wanted me to be angry (it was good for me). Gregory cried for himself and me. Carmen tried to comfort me and said that I would pull through it; she would help me. Wila offered to do anything she could, to take me places, to care for me. Rosalind, my predecessor on the cancer path, whom I had regularly visited during her hospitalization for chemotherapy, offered me comforting words with the serenity of one who had descended to Hades and was able to talk about it. Other friends offered what they could, all of them revealing, in this unplanned test of confrontation with a death threat, their Rorschachlike responses of caring and willingness to help.

Jaunary 19

On the afternoon when I called Dr. Marcus, I also called Dr. Carter, my internist of several years. He reacted in his usual distant way. He was sorry. Then, like a minister reciting the final prayers before a burial, without changing the monotone of a routine service, because for him the corpse was a routine corpse, he listed my advantages in facing the cancer: 1) I was in general good health; 2) detection was early; 3) nowadays treatment is very successful. Finally he asked a question, rhetorically, that he promptly answered himself. Could he help me in any way? No, he couldn't. This was a surgical matter, and only the surgeon could help. When he stopped talking I knew that this conversation was our last. I don't know if he knew it too, that from now on my internist would be my oncologist. I felt let down, sad, hoping that he would give some indication of compassion, of concern for a patient he had seen for years. I knew his habit of dictating a note at once. I fantasized, using magical thinking to induce him to do it, that he would dictate a note wishing me well. For a few days I actually hoped to find a two-line note from him in my mail. I did not. He never obeyed my mental command. So we parted forever over my breast cancer, without words and without tears. My tears I cried alone. I was terribly sad. No matter how old and mature and knowledgeable we are, a doctor is always a parental protector, someone who must care for us. I felt neglected, insignificant, irrelevant, just one more patient in his practice. The *me* who had been so tried those days felt the pain of a neglect that could have been avoided by two or three simple words on a white piece of paper or even on the telephone: "I wish you well," or any other equivalent. Their absence was like a suction, emptying years of a professional relationship into an ending without human emotional contact. I did not want to lose Dr. Carter that way, that is, by his letting me go to so terrible a medical encounter without a kind word.

The weekend stretched into infinitely long hours, very long days. My friends called me one after the other, invited me to dinner, took me to the movies, told me jokes, feasted me with sweets and delicacies. I could enjoy them only a bit. The tension of waiting was like walking a tightrope.

On Sunday afternoon, a joyful voice greeted me when I answered the phone. It was Nino Carolli, who had come from Italy to participate in a scientific meeting in New York. He had flown from Rome and was full of exciting feelings. I tried not to dampen his joy, but I could not help using the only voice I had, funereal and cracking with suppressed sobs. He became alarmed. Immediately I found myself telling him the whole truth. Then we both were on the point of tears. We decided that the best thing would be for him to come to dinner at my house – he could help me cook – so that I could talk without being ashamed of having my face covered with tears. He came, and we cooked, chatted, ate, and cried all at the same time. His very presence consoled me. To be able to talk from the heart, honestly crying as much as one needs, with a friend one respects and loves is a rare privilege. We were as sad as we could be, but we were at peace in the sharing of honest and undisguised pain. We agreed that he would call me from New York to learn the news. We embraced and he left, burdened with my pain. I started feeling sad for having spoiled his visit to the States but consoled and content for having shared with him my fright and having experienced his true affection for me. When he left, *me* had returned to her highest level of dignified pain, self-respect, and even sense of humor. I was beginning to see that the state of *me* at this terrible juncture depended, as though I were a little child, on the respect and the attention paid to me by friends. I also needed to know that the other person cared more about *me* than about my cancer. I could not help laughing when I noticed that I, that is *me*, was jealous of my cancer. I did not want my cancer to be more important than I was myself. Nino's greatest gesture of friendship was to show that he was a friend of *me*.

The cancer had also infiltrated my sense of self, shattering my self-assured feeling that I was in possession of myself. The delicate, smooth integration of the machinery that makes "me" was screeching at every turn. I was many. I was I, the one who tried so desperately to remain in charge. And then there were all the other "me's": the one who wanted to remain the same, the "me" changed by cancer, the "me" who wanted to die, and the "me" who wanted to live. Suddenly, in less than two weeks, I had become an unruly crowd of simultaneously needy and proud "me's," each pleading for respect, attention, and tender care.

Monday came and went, with patients and paper work and a terrible silence from the doctors. There was no news. I repeated, like an old woman mumbling Hail Marys on her rosary beads, "Dr. Robbins said he'd call on Monday or Tuesday." Tuesday came, and I blessed my patients because they had long ago obtained from me a commitment that I would attend to them and their feelings regardless of my own feelings. I had to force myself to do it, but I did it as a soldier carries out his orders even if he is shaking in his boots.

In the late afternoon I sat next to the phone and tried to read. An early call at 4:00 P.M. spared me long hours of pretending. Dr. Robbins said, in his firm and slightly cheerful but matter-of-fact voice, that the pathologist had confirmed that the cancer was invasive and that based on the cells' morphology and their invasiveness a mastectomy should be the treatment of choice. I asked him if he had asked the pathologist to send the slides to Dr. Nagle and his pathologist for a second opinion. He said he had. I immediately called Dr. Nagle, who had seen the slides. He too recommended a mastectomy for two reasons: 1) the invasiveness already present would require a large lumpectomy followed by radiation and 2) that there was a risk of other cancerous areas in the rest of the breast. Then, after mastectomy, if I had no metastasis, I would probably not need chemotherapy.

I had independently decided that I did not want radiation. The risk of complications seemed high for me in spite of what Dr. Hughes had said. Besides, once complications appeared, the consequences could be severe and irreversible. I asked a few more questions. Then we both agreed that I should have a mastectomy. Dr. Nagle said that I had to have bone, liver, and lung scans before the surgery. Without wasting a second, I called Dr. Robbins back and asked him if he could perform the operation on December 22 (when I was supposed to be in the Caribbean). He said that he had already scheduled the operating room for my surgery. Then I told him about the scans Dr. Nagle had requested. He said he was going to arrange for me to have them all in two days, between Wednesday and Friday. Surgery was scheduled for Monday. It was now 4:00 P.M. on the preceding Tuesday. A few minutes later his secretary called, telling me to report the following day for a preadmission workup. She then would meet me there and tell me the times of the other appointments.

I had to juggle my patients' schedules to make room for my own medical care. A couple of patients had to change their own days to accommodate me. One could not make it. We canceled. It was just four days before my scheduled vacation, and I could see that these last four days, already worrisome for them because of my impending absence, would now become frenetic for me and disturbing to those entrusted to my care. It was obvious to me that no matter how hard I tried, I could not help hurting some of them. I found myself limited in my ability to be emotionally available to their pain, their frustrations, or their wishes to punish me for taking a vacation. I tried as hard as I could to forgive myself for a limitation that was beyond my human capacity. I hoped that in their ignorance of my misery, my patients could forgive me for failing them.

January 20

Wednesday, Thursday, and Friday were among the most frantic days of my entire life. To have all the tests performed, I had to go back and forth to the hospital three times a day. I had to rush out of the office the moment a patient left, dash to the hospital, and announce, "I only have 75 minutes because a patient is waiting for me." In my comings and goings I functioned with the precision of a Swiss train, my eyes fixed on my watch. I could not cancel the patients without their suspecting that there was something really the matter with me. Besides, I had already told my Monday patients that I had to move my vacation up one day and that I would see them on Saturday. One patient refused to make the change and missed one hour, an hour she badly needed. In spite of it all, I tried to listen, but I simply could not. I did not want to think about anybody else but me.

The bone scan brought new fears to my already frightened disposition. The technician who did the bone scan said kindly but seriously that I needed more X-rays of the pelvis and of my left leg because there was something unusual there. I became *certain* that I had pelvic metastasis and gave myself a few months to leave this world. I felt terribly sad and even imagined myself crippled by diffuse metastatic illness. I found myself crying, discreet tears trembling on my eyelashes. After minutes as long as eons, the doctor came out saying he had to talk with me. I spoke to him with the imperative voice of a judge in court, "Tell me yes or no. Do *I* have metastasis?" He fired back: "No, no you don't." "Fine," I said. "That is fine." Then he posed *his* problem to me.

I was delighted *he* had a *problem* even if it was about my bones. He said he could not make sense of the fact that my right sacroiliac joint had collected more radioactive material than the left side. He asked me if I had pain there or any known trouble. After much searching he found satisfaction in learning that I limp on my left leg and that therefore my right leg carries more weight. Now he could write a meaningful report. We parted as relaxed friends.

The following day I died a similar death. The technician carried out the procedures for the liver scan. Then he asked me to wait until the doctor saw it. He returned and, with what seemed to me a mournful face, asked me to return for more scanning of my liver. This time, I decided, it was the real thing: I *did* have liver metastasis. My father's mother had died at 53 – my age – of liver cancer. It was only fitting that I, her granddaughter, follow suit. I saw myself, yellow, icteric, with dry skin, skeletonlike, with a gigantic belly, like a malnourished child with bulging sad eyes, dying of liver cancer. I felt terribly sorry for myself and my ugly death. While I was "dying," the technician asked me to wait in a private waiting room, which I immediately decided was the chamber of deadly announcements for victims of terminal cancer. After a very long time the doctor came out and introduced himself and said he had to talk with me. This time I mumbled like a beggar who has not eaten in three days, "Please, do I have metastasis?"

He quickly said, "No. Oh no, certainly not!"

"Thank you," I said, interrupting him, and it was one of the most sincere "thank yous" I have said in my life.

He too had a problem. My left liver lobe had some scarring he had to account for. I – free of metastasis – joyfully informed him that I had had hepatitis-A as a child and hepatitis-B at age 40. He found my report of hepatitis compatible with the liver scan abnormalities. He said that, as a doctor, he had to make me aware of my liver damage. I thanked him for his concern even though I wanted to hug him for having found in me *only* a scarred left liver lobe.

Finally I had to go to the dentist to get protection for my upper teeth during the intubation for the anesthetic. I also had to give my own blood in case I should need a transfusion after surgery. At the blood bank I felt like a leper, because of my two bouts with hepatitis, my blood had to be marked DANGEROUS, not usable by anybody else. The head nurse, who drew my blood, was very kind and concerned and told me about a close friend who had lost the battle against cancer and could die that very night. Her eyes welled up while she said that her friend had found great serenity in facing death. I felt I had been invited to join the Sacred Order of the Dying and that it was my privilege now to hear the sorrows of those acquainted with death. She and I talked quietly and softly about the acceptance of death. We had a rare moment of human intimacy in which we shared her sorrow at her young friend's impending death and my sorrow at my encounter with the deadly threat of cancer. The serenity she beautifully described as coloring her dying friend's last days enveloped our encounter in the way the mist of summer rain envelops a garden. We parted as friends, ready for the sad days to come.

January 25

The fear of death and deadly illness that gripped me during that fateful week had prompted me to forget my encounter with the plastic surgeon, who had announced life after surgery and the possibility of my having the semblance of a normal breast. On Tuesday, two days before the scans, late in the afternoon, after my talk with Drs. Robbins and Nagle, I met with the plastic surgeon in his office in the hospital basement. Dr. Keily was a tall, gracious, well-mannered man who spoke to me respectfully and with the tone of voice and modulation of someone who is aware of another person's great sorrow. He created a relaxed atmosphere before we spoke together about my breasts, knowing that in a week's time my right breast would be gone. He measured me and my breasts, asked questions, showed me surgical means of breast reconstruction and of breast implants. I immediately said that I had had too much surgery in my life to want another procedure that would require tearing under from the back or the abdomen to shape a breast. I questioned him about the implants. A certain joy came upon him when he showed me "the implant" and "the expander." He was like a mature child who loved playing with those lovely plastic shapes, like balloons for grownups.

He explained that "the expander" (a round plastic bag with a tube called "the port") could be placed under the pectoral muscle immediately after the mastectomy, during the same operation. Then he would use "the port" to inject saline solution to expand the skin progressively. When the bag and the skin over it had reached the size of the other breast, he would remove the expander and place "the implant" there for good. The implant, a tea-colored plastic mass with the consistency of a real breast, was now in my hand. I touched it, moved it from side to side and tossed it between my hands as though I liked the breast shape. I imagined it under my skin, a fake breast, a plastic breast for me, a person just about to become a civilized bionic woman of sorts. I was trying to put distance, comic distance, between myself and what was to come. Such banality in the horror of it all: while my breast of flesh was awaiting there, helpless and marked for surgical destruction, I was playing, pitifully content, with the hideous and appealing plastic breast. I felt hatred, despair, and immense fatigue in the absurdity of the moment. I tried to return to my rational self and asked Dr. Keily all the questions that occurred to me about complications, infections, adverse reaction, and related matters. We talked about each of them until I was satisfied that it was a safe procedure. Still, I needed more time, particularly in a moment of such great inner turmoil, to be able to decide if I preferred to have plastic surgery or simply to have my scar, to acknowledge that I was a maimed woman wearing a post-mastectomy bra.

Dr. Keily was in no hurry. He said, "Think about it. Call me, or come if you want to. You can decide just before surgery. I'll go to see you before you go in. If you want to, I can make a few marks on your chest for Dr. Robbins to see what I need for my surgery."

Dr. Keily's relaxed and quietly content manner brought a different note to my frantic march toward a mastectomy. Without saying it, he was talking about my everyday future, my going places comfortably, sure that I looked as though I had two breasts. He spoke of living as an ordinary woman, the simple life of attending to clothes, looks, bathing suits, and bras. The visit was like a little oasis of life in a desert of desolation and death. I felt gratitude and a childish wish to cling to him, to make him the only one to deal with me, as though by his offering me his toy breasts I would not have to lose my real one.

There was nothing else to do. Dr. Robbins called to set up the final details. I had to report to day surgery at 10:30 A.M. on Monday, December 22, bringing with me as little as possible. From that moment on they would take care of me. First they would operate on me. Then I would go to the recovery room and when fully awake go to my room. I was not to eat anything after midnight of the previous day.

Now that I had consented to my fate, there was nothing medical left to do. It was time to face the whole implication of the event for my life. I had been debating whether to inform a few relatives I have abroad or to leave them uninformed and tell them later. I decided that it was too risky to go for surgery without telling them. I could die, even if the risk was small. Besides, I was going to be out of commission for some time if I had metastasis, and I could not lie to them. I also knew that calling meant upsetting their lives and confronting them with the impotence of the immense distance between us. I knew that they could not bridge the distance. I called my cousin Bryant, who immediately wanted to come but realized that he had neither a valid passport nor a visa and that it takes a long time to get a visa. He then asked me many questions. I gave him the phone number of a friend who would keep him informed. A few days before calling my cousin, I had called my good friends Maria, Fabio, and Jacinta, all in Spain. Jacinta had had a bilateral mastectomy. At that time she had called me, and I had consulted on her behalf with some of the top experts in this country. They were now my doctors. We spoke together for a long time, two women sharing their pain, their fears, and their courage, conveying tenderness and care through 5,000 miles of telephone wires. I felt that Jacinta, like Beatrice who led Dante in his celestial travels, was guiding me with equal gentleness through the labyrinth of feeling evoked by the land of breast cancer.

February 1

Now I had to wait until Monday for the surgery. An unexpected serenity came upon me, like the calm after a storm has devastated a landscape. Every fiber in me had been shaken, battered, stretched to the limit by the forcefulness of the wind storm. And, now, there on the horizon, arching over the broken branches, a barely visible rainbow appeared. It was, like the first rainbow, a sign of accepting peace, of submission to my condition of not owning my own life, of facing the risk of beginning again when the murderous waters come down. Perhaps it was also the feeling Noah must have felt: in a sea of death his ark was still supported on the surface of life by the killer of all other living creatures. It was a good feeling of wonder and hope, of foreboding and horror. The hour of doves had not yet come.

Life *had* to go on. I decided to go to a lecture and reception I had been invited to. It was important to me. I wanted to meet people from the new faculty I had just joined.

I was acutely aware of being divided between my precancer self – curious, excitable, eager to be there in the midst of life – and this new, cancerous me, afraid of death and desolation, a me on the way out of the celebration of life. Nobody noticed anything. I did not want anybody to notice. I engaged with passion in a discussion with a professor of Greek culture about Oedipus's and Jocasta's attitude toward the truth.

On Saturday I saw my patients until early afternoon. After a rest, I returned to the office to leave everything in order: the billing done, the correspondence answered, the filing done, as I usually do before a vacation.

On Sunday I went to High Mass, and while the choir was singing the alleluia I transported my imagined postdead self into the presence of my Maker and wished I would be granted the grace of finding all the creatures of this vast universe, big and small, singing the alleluia of life in their diverse, tiny or thunderous voices. I felt for a moment the atemporality, the weightlessness of my imagined eternity. I also real-ized that I was incapable of imagining myself as simply not being. I, while I was, was in fact immortal. I smiled, thinking how right good old Freud had been in saying that the unconscious harbors no notion of death. The alleluia was coming to an end, after having opened for me a broad Jacob's ladder between heaven and earth.

Then a friend and I went to lunch; we both felt entitled to a true gourmet treat. Finally, I got home and prepared everything to take to the hospital. Gregory and Carmen were to take me in the morning to the hospital. A dear child, Linda, the daughter of very close friends from high school days, was to come with me to the hospital. As a second year medical student, she hoped to be permitted to stay with me until the moment of the operation. She was most tender and most proud. She was experiencing the fullness of having grown up and having entered the secret chambers of the adults. In her compassionate companionship there was also the sense that she was participating from inside in the journey between life and death that any surgical operation takes the patient through. Her shining face and intelligent dark eyes modulated in their beaming youthfulness the gloom of my voluntary maiming. She was bursting with life, with the joy of seeing herself growing into a competent physician capable of wresting victims out of the jaws of death. There I was, lying naked on the stretcher, a white sheet over my body. I was coming as a supplicant for life, offering my breast as a propitiatory gift to the hungry goddess of cancer. Like the devout Aztecs, I was willing to place on her altar the palpitating organ that would save the life of the people.

Then, one by one, dressed like comically grotesque characters in a children's play, nurses and doctors came to render their services to me. I, a naked queen in the wonderland of surgery, held court with them, consenting, requesting, warning, asking for faithful services to my precious person. They all behaved gently, speaking with modulated voices full of concern equidistant between technical efficiency and emotional contact with me.

The plastic surgeon came to see whether I wanted the euphemistically named "expander" to start my breast replacement. I agreed, and we proceeded to sign the consent form. Then came the anesthetist, who started the I.V. and questioned me extensively to be sure that the procedure would be as safe as possible. Finally, came Dr. Robbins, who with his contained cheerfulness asked me how I was. I told him the truth. "I wish I could say I am well, but I am sad and frightened. However," I said, perhaps competing a little with his cheerfulness, "I still have my wits about me." He put his hand on my hand and patted it a little as though he knew, naturally, that my façade of trying to remain the mature woman I am did not fully hide the scared child in need of holding and parental protection.

Linda kissed me and left, and I was wheeled into the operating room. They asked me to move onto the operating table. I could see them all dressed in green, surrounding me in a circle, only their eyes visible. I could see their concentration on the task, their becoming progressively a technical team to do their work on me. I could also see that they cared. But I could not help being afraid of their terrible tools for cutting and maiming. When the anesthetist announced to me, "Dr. Meldin, in a few minutes you'll be fully asleep," I pleaded humbly to them, trying to appeal to their highest sense of medical responsibility, "Into your hands I entrust my anatomy." After that I was a dream in a body that was being maimed.

February 8

Opening my eyes, I returned from the land of merciful anesthesia and saw three smiling faces, eyes shining. They were making cooing sounds as though I were a baby waking from a long sleep or perhaps a sleeping beauty of sorts who needed to be invited, gently but firmly, to return to the land of the waking people. Blanche, my good friend from adolescent days, was there now, holding my hand. Linda, her medical student daughter, and Tom, her son, were with her, cheering me on with their offerings: roses, a fluffy toy dog, and a Snoopy balloon exclaiming, "Get Well!" There was another one saying, "Happy Birthday!" because the death of my right breast had coincided with the day I had entered this world. At that time I was very well made, with every organ in place in a wonderful, functional body preprogrammed with precise mechanisms for my entire life. Today, in the 54th year of my well-running organism, I had had to offer up my breast, a part of myself, to save my whole self.

I kept my sad thoughts to myself. I could see that Blanche, Linda, and Tom desperately wanted to comfort me, to console me, to make me feel that I was my good old self, breast or no breast. They said it in every way it could be said, mostly with their genuine presence, their unspoken message that I, though humiliated and shaky, was the one they loved, recognized, and cared for. Once they saw that I was not in acute pain and that I still had my wits about me, they introduced, as if on tiptoe, the delightful, playful good humor we always shared. When they saw me laughing, they began to laugh too, almost giggling, as children do when they have been very scared and the moment of relief comes.

I felt tremendous gratitude for their presence. There was nothing I needed more than that: very familiar faces, faces to rest my eyes, my wishes, my fears on without having to select what to show and what to hide. Resting on the face of another is the deepest feeling of trust I am able to experience. It must be what infants feel when they need to see their mothers' face. I, like a swaddled infant, rested my sleepy eyes on my friends' gentle faces and fell asleep until the next morning.

I was awakened very early by the residents and attendants making rounds. They encircled my bed and with sincere and cheerful voices exclaimed, after carefully checking me, that I was doing splendidly well. There was no bleeding, no fever, no complications, only a bit of pain, and the nurses had reported that "the patient rested well." They congratulated me for my success and asked me if I wanted to know anything or ask any questions. I wanted to say, "I want my breast back." Instead I asked about moving a little and about the condition of my arm, because they had posted an enormous sign saying, "No venipunctures or blood pressure on Dr. Meldin's right arm." It had the looks of a medieval edict posted for the execution of a criminal.

Dr. Murray, the resident in plastic surgery answered, and the team agreed, "You arm should be perfectly all right. However, we have removed the lymph nodes, and it should be protected. You can move it a little. You can move your hand as much as you want." They wished me a good day and left, content with me, their patient who had given them the medical satisfaction of recovering according to the prescribed patterns of a surgical postmastectomy course. I was surprised to experience a paradoxical feeling of pride at seeing them leave self-satisfied with their competence. It was a feeling of having done my homework well or having set the table properly for my mother, as if I were a six-year-old girl who had behaved well and felt entitled to a little bit of love and praise.

The rounds were to take place every morning as an early liturgy of hospital awakening. I noticed that we were becoming "ten minutes in the morning friends," and I was beginning to look forward to their collective visits. We seemed to be pleased with each other in a mild version of a mutual admiration society. They kept me as well as possible in my sorrowful condition, and I, the patient, satisfied their sense of mastery by having my body behave as they medicated it. All things going well, we liked each other. I, the anguished and disrupted I, had no complaints about them. Their compassionate, matter-of-fact approach served me well. I needed my dignity and my adult self to provide a sanctuary of silent reverence for me to mourn my breast, to face the horror of possible protracted illness, and the stark aloneness of death. I also needed that sanctuary to search within me for the wellsprings of life. Cancer tolerates no lies. Preachments do not

console the victim. Superficial encouragement betrays the integrity of
the knowledge that cancer is an unmistakable threat to personal life.
Surgery removes the main source, the deadly spring of fast footed
colonizing cells. Chemotherapy, an internal atom bomb, blasts any
cell, malignant or innocent, caught in the forbidden act of reproduc-
tion. Words and platitudes do not touch the center of life from which
we live. Surgery and chemotherapy destroy the source of death. Blind
as they both are to the microscopic bearers of bad tidings, they can
never certify that they have seen the last metastatic cell die. The most
advanced technical devices we have today have to rely on the most
ancient human helper: hope. They have to hope that they have killed
every cell. The life of a person depends on that killing, but they still
have to *hope* they were killed. Beyond their hope is the cancerous cells'
fierce determination to live, to grow, and to multiply.

"To search for the wellsprings of life," I thought in my long hours
crying in bed with convalescent fatigue, "I have to find something in
me, something true, genuine, honest to God and me, that wanted life.
Cancer tolerates no lies. No one can do it but me. No one can promise
that if I find the secret place from which life enters in me , I will be able
to use it, to contain the disruptions in my body that allowed the
cancer to grow."

The existential paradox of being human confronted me with its
unshakable finality. We inhabit a body that must die, sooner or later,
and we have no ruling power over the fragile house in which we live.
"The best we can do," I thought in my pondering search, "is to live in
peace, in true, profound, integrated peace in our home, this earthen-
ware house that comes from the dust and returns to the dust. If there
is to be hope for me, there has to be peace. True, integrated, shared,
realistic peace has to be there. That peace requires wide open eyes,
acceptance of the full reality of the threat of cancer and also a
self-assured conviction that in life and death I, myself, am more than
my cancer and my death."

This discovery, made in between concerns about eating, bowel
movements, exercises, and multisided conversations with friends who
flocked to my bedside, did not solve the problem. The search had to go
on, perhaps for months, perhaps for years. The discovery of a small
lump on my right breast had dislodged me from my existential
complacency. Now, like a medieval pilgrim, a searcher for the Holy
Grail, a mendicant for the face of God, an itinerant stumbling on the

path to the wellsprings of life, I had begun a journey along the meandering roads of meaning. "Meaning," the Zen master said, "is there where you are fully where you are."

So in between hospital routines of changing dressings and pulling tubes, moving bowels and tossing sleepless in bed, I, in my weakened body, started the secret journey to the unnamed place the Zen master had pointed to. "This journey," I read, "you have to make alone." So it was and is, and I think, now that I write about it, so it will be. In being born and in dying we are alone. From now on, I began to understand, I had to live my everyday life with its every delightful and annoying detail, while trying to advance, in darkness and in light, on the road to uncompromising meaning.

I also became a pilgrim in the many corridors of the hospital ward. The doctors recommended that I walk and exercise my arm to help the recovery. It was the oncology war. Looking at all of us, some young people, half eaten by cancer, some courageous, terminally ill old gentlemen, and others, I recalled the 23rd psalm: "The Lord is my shepherd. . . . Even though I walk in the valley of the dead I shall not fear." But I felt fear, the fear of death, of protracted illness, of losing mastery over my life. I was aware that I was waiting for the pathologist's report about my lymph nodes revealing whether or not there was the presence of ominous metastasis. If it was present, then I would join those who walk in the valley of the dead.

I walked around and around to bring my stamina back. I dared myself to face the self-consciousness of walking around in a long robe, revealing the unevenness of my one breasted chest. I felt that that was a necessary act of honesty to my fellow patients and to myself, an act of factual, if painful, acceptance.

I also exercised my arm under the direction of the nurse, who commanded, "You must loosen up your shoulder joint. Bend down and make a circle as wide as possible, letting gravity play a part in the movement." I did. "Good," she said. "Now," she ordered, "walk the wall with your fingers as high above your head as you can." Well, I could not do much. She understood that it was just the beginning of my "walking walls" with my fingers. She continued with stern compassion, "You *must* do it several times a day until you have full range of movement; otherwise you will have a stiff shoulder." So I walked my arm up and down, like a kindergartener playing a vertical piece on a hospital room wall.

Everyone approved of me as a "good" patient when the time for release came. My discharge summary glowed with superlatives. "Dr. Meldin is doing splendidly well," "marvelous cicatrization," "no complications." " 'Summa cum laude' in mastectomy," I thought, noticing the paradox between tragedy and glory.

3 ❧

Home Survival

Febuary 15

The time for discharge was drawing near. Being a woman alone, I had to plan for the handling of my house by others. Like the captain of a small vessel who has to promote the second mate to officer in charge, I had to hire someone for a while to help me with the chores I would not be able to do until full recovery. Thus I entered another unknown universe, that of agencies for household help. I learned in a brief period of time that good home care and good home helpers are as rare as diamonds. One agency after the other promised help but failed—at the last minute—to provide it. I learned that those who do come and help are women on the edges of society. They move from state to state with their fatherless children on their own pilgrimage to scratch out a living with temporary work. They come from marginal immigrant groups and have a private network of connections, a subterranean tunnel of communication, to get jobs. They stay for a while and then disappear, pulled by some private tragedy, some restless need to change, some hope for betterment elsewhere, or perhaps attracted by a new hope for love and a loving man. Five of them (all of them black) came and went, impressing me with their intelligence, their good will, their eagerness to earn money, and their great secrecy about themselves and their lives. Each in turn disappeared into nowhere. Disappointed as I was, because I had begun to like each woman and her work, I felt a tremendous compassion for this flock of women besieged by poverty and instability, unable in their complex circumstances to grow roots in their environment. I discovered in each woman one of my neighbors whom I had not yet met, as the Gospels say. It was a paradox. I, who should have been the Samaritan, needed the help of those who had been left on the wayside of life. I noticed that I was learning too many paradoxes in too brief a time. "Well," I thought, "such is the school of life and death."

Two days after my discharge and eight days after the surrendering of my breast, Dr. Robbins called, and this time his voice was not cheerful. He said, "There are two lymph nodes with metastatic cancer cells. It is not as bad as it seems," he continued hurriedly. "The lymph nodes are proximal, the closest to the breast." I had not much to say. Such facts are so rotund and weighty that they require no questions. He continued, "In the past we did not recommend chemotherapy for only two nodes ['Only two nodes!' I shouted internally], but experience has proven that chemotherapy *prolongs* [I noticed the word 'prolongs'] life. Today we even use it in cases when there is no metastasis. You and Dr. Nagle should decide about it. Chemotherapy is my recommendation." I asked him how soon it could be started. He said not before four to six weeks after surgery. The body had to take time to recover. Besides, Dr. Nagle and I had to decide what was the best combination of drugs for me, given my age and the type of cancer I had.

I became acutely aware that I had taken a new path into the valley of the dead and that what Dr. Robbins and I had said in our conversation closed the surgical gate and opened the gate that leads to chemical warfare with cancer. The war by removal of the enemy had been won. Now the oncologist and I had to kill the remaining infiltrators and terrorists who could come from their minuscule hideaways and assault me by surprise and do me in at the moment I least expected it. From now on, like a nation besieged by infiltrators, I and my doctors had to live a vigilant life and create a C.I.A. for an internal survey of undesirable murderers. I needed this comparison, this politically distancing description with all the euphemisms of the press, to bear the sheer terror of the death installed in my flesh.

My body had become a dangerous cavern that could harbor in its recesses – hidden and well kept – my worst enemies. A political battle against fierce insurrection had begun. Those for the nation, the doctors and I, allied in the efforts to exterminate the enemy, would have to kill criminals and bystanders alike "for the good of the nation." We would have to kill the cancerous cells *and* each normal unsuspecting cell in my body caught by the chemical in the unforgivable act of reproducing. The cells so found would be summarily executed, the innocent also dying so that the criminals would be eradicated in the massacre. The method of Herod is today called in medical terminology "chemotherapy," and I consented to it.

Three weeks later, the oncologist and I, two thoughtful doctors weighing facts, publications, statistics, death and survival charts, side effects, and results graphs, decided on the standard source of chemotherapy: CMF, the elegant consonants for three deadly drugs, Cytoxan, Methotrexate, and 5-fluoruracil, euphemistically called a cocktail for breast cancer, a well-studied bombastic combination with the best results. I did not yet have the courage to talk about prognosis. I felt I had to bite one bullet first and then start thinking about the facts – not only the fears – of life and death.

I had all the tests. I was fit to start the uneven war. The date was set for seven weeks after the surgery, the explanations given. The nurse who was to be my nurse for the course of the eight treatments I was to have, came in. She was a young pregnant woman, smiling and obviously very poised when dealing with nervous wrecks like myself. Her name was Monique. She told me that we would stay together, explained the mechanics of the procedures, gave me stickers for the parking lot (now that I was a regular, I had the right to some privileges), and set up a time and a day for my first I.V. infusion as an outpatient. She told me I could drive home myself because the side effects would not appear until after four hours following the injection of the chemicals. So we parted from each other allies for a six-month war, the time it would take to give me eight treatments at three-week intervals.

February 22

There was a waiting period until the first injection. I had been told, as I had known, that I would lose my hair and need a wig.

I looked in the yellow pages, and much to my amazement I found a vast array of stores providing every wig imaginable. Like Alice, I had found another surprise in the Wonderland of Cancer. They advertised bluntly: "Wigs for chemotherapy patients and other hair problems. Discretion. Efficiency. Call today." Rosalind, my friend of many years, had gone through the same thing with her own cancer. She recommended the Italian man who had made her second wig and who knew the art of consoling her in her bald despair. Alexander mentioned a shop in the neighborhood whose owner, a woman, had helped a relative of his. Both Rosalind and Alexander insisted that I make sure I get a wig that I truly liked, a wig that would make me feel myself. I was moved because they seemed to understand so well that "me" had to be protected with respectful and adequate care.

I had always taken my hair for granted. My hair is unusual. Thin and silky with large natural waves, it has never required any other care than a good shampoo and a comb and brush to acquire a becoming shape. The only trouble was to find a hair dresser who knew how to cut hair that was intent in going its own way. Several years ago I found Daniel, a thin, tall black man, who expertly set out to get me the perfect cut. Since the day of our meeting, Daniel and I had been greatly satisfied with each other, and I, relying on the skill of his scissored hands, had long forgotten my worries.

Now I had to start all over again and find someone who would make a wig that looked like my unusual hair. Childhood memories rushed back to add worries to my worries. When I was four years old I was left in the care of my grandaunt and aunt. They were to get me ready for the return of my parents, who would take my brother and me to an outing. I was all ready, feeling quite elegant with my ribboned white dress and patent leather shoes, my pocketbook, my gloves, and a felt hat matching my dress. All I needed was to have my hair combed. My grandaunt made me stand on a bathroom stool and started to brush and comb my hair, but my hair had a will of its own. She wanted it to go one way, but it wanted to go another way. After trying every bit of knowledge she had about taming a strand of hair, she called in despair to my aunt Tota. With self-assured confidence, my aunt started the task of making my hair pretty. She sprayed my hair with a bit of water to help out, but humidity only increased my hair's self-determined tendencies to curl in its own way. My aunt was at her wit's end when my mother came. My mother had figured out something very simple: let my hair go its own way. Like a savior of a desolate child and two afflicted women, and in only a few seconds, she combed my hair and her fingers encouraged my curls to do what they wanted. In three minutes my head looked, so they said, like Shirley Temple's. I felt the very proud child of a knowledgeable mother who had rescued me at the last minute.

The story returned now as an omen, announcing unforeseen difficulties and unfulfillable tasks. I decided to call and ask questions until I had the courage to make an appointment. I found the courage by acknowledging to myself that in a few weeks I was going to be bald like an inmate of some *gulag*.

The male voice that answered the first call was full, caressing, and encouraging. It had acquired the perfect professional touch to deal with human pain. I was a bit seduced and a great deal relieved. The man explained that he would make me a natural hair wig, an exact match of my own color and texture, and that he was delighted to see me for a free consultation. He said I could come right away. So I went as I was, wearing my household clothes.

His shop had two parts. One was for ordinary people who needed a regular beauty parlor. The other, behind innocent screens, opened into a large room whose walls were covered with shelves. At the end there was a small parlor for the patients who came in shame to cover their baldness.

A clerk graciously asked me a few questions and offered me a cup of coffee. I had to wait a little for Leon, the man in charge, the owner of the caressing voice. Coffee cup in hand, I turned to look around. A hundred styrofoam heads, male and female, facelessly white, covered by every imaginable hair style, encompassing every racial group—straight, thick, black, Chinese parted hair, radiantly bright red Irish curls—rested on the shelves.

Alice herself, poised as she was in her Wonderland explorations, would have been startled by the eyeless staring of the bodiless faces. Anger, despair, sadness came upon me. I felt I was in a funerary chamber and that each of those heads was waiting there with the certainty of a murderer for the person who, sentenced to death, would need that hair to cover the shame of having been already made bald as a preparation for the final blow. Words of indignation came to me. I addressed the wig forms in my mind as though they could understand me. "You," I said, "You prophets of doom, you evil spirits, you just wait there with your calm certainty that the victim will come. You, you, and you, I hate you, each and every one of you. I hate that you can wait, still and unfeeling, wearing the hair that despairing men and women would fetch from you to cover their shame. I despise you."

They did not respond. The Alice in me was both disappointed and relieved because, deep down in that recess of myself where I was trembling, I knew I needed them, and it would not have been good for me if the one I needed had refused to surrender her hair.

Leon came in and, like a well-trained doctor, chatted with me and put me at my ease, and like a good Italian told me twice that with my pretty face any wig would do. My good humor, thanks to his protective manner, returned to me. I retorted, "Do not say it once more because I may believe it." We both laughed, and the laughter sealed a friendly alliance to go on with the sessions of finding me a good wig. We listed assets and problems: type of hair, ways of keeping the wig on my head, the care of it, the pros and the cons of everything. Then we started trying on the wigs.

The mirror began to reflect new versions of me. Each wig was a new variation, up to now indistinguishable, of what I could look like with this hairdo and that hairdo. I oscillated between fascination, a sense of adventure, and a stubborn feeling that welled up from my deepest recesses. Finally, the feeling found a voice. "I," I said, "I want to look like *myself*." Leon understood. He asked, now like a well-trained psychiatrist, what would make me feel like *me*.

I said that I wanted to keep my forehead free of hair. I wanted soft hair. I wanted to keep the smallness of my head as it was, all the wigs were too big for me. He said soothingly, "Don't you worry. We can do that easily. We'll measure your head. We'll take photographs of how it is now, and we'll make you a wig that replicates your head as closely as possible. All that people may think—if they do—is that you have set your hair more carefully. Trust us; we are experts. We *will* help you."

I felt like throwing my arms around his neck and kissing him. Instead I said, "I am very grateful, Leon, that you exist and that you have this store. You make a great difference in a moment like this." He soberly said that he understood and proceeded to make me try on two more wigs. One of them was like a miracle. I saw *me* in the mirror. I almost shouted, "That is me, Leon!" He smiled knowingly and said, "I told you we would find a wig for you." I felt relieved, almost elated. I got hold of a mirror and checked that I looked like *me* from every angle of vision. It was not quite perfect, but Leon expertly said he could fix this and he could fix that. Then he modulated my enthusiasm at having found a "me wig." "Do not make a decision now," he said. "Go home and think about more questions, and then come back and we will start the work. You still have time. It takes a few weeks before your hair falls out, and you have not yet started the chemotherapy," he said knowingly.

It made sense. Then it occurred to me that it would be better to come with a friend who could look more objectively at the whole process. He agreed that that was an excellent idea. I was to call in a few days. We parted friends and partners in the task of covering my imminent baldness.

March 1

Now to find the right friend to help me assess the "me wig." I thought of Carmen, who knew me so well. She was busy, though, and would have to leave her work. Besides, her pain over my illness was intense even when she covered it up. Her sister had died of breast cancer. I thought of Rosalind, my friend with cancer. I felt compassion for both of us and decided that it was too much to ask of her to go again through the memories of her own suffering with wigs. Suddenly it occurred to me that a young woman at the highest point of her coquettish seductiveness would be the best judge in this matter of beauty and self-concern.

I called Linda, my young friend, the medical student who was with me before surgery. I had known her very well all of her 27 years, and I had watched with pleasure her growth from the time she was crawling in diapers to the present. She had become a poised young woman, bright eyed with the excitement of life, love, and knowledge. We had moved from a relationship of "aunt," the friend of her parents, to being personal friends. We were now in the habit of discussing the deepest matters of the heart: love, men, life issues, and God him/herself. I had learned to enjoy the sunny warmth of her youthful zest for life, while she seemed to find a measure of safety in her actions by discussing with me her visions and findings.

I called Linda and asked her if she was willing to be the surveyor and custodian of my hair looks. She was elated. For her, she said, it was to enter a new world she had never imagined. She promised to be careful and strict in her judgment and guaranteed that under her careful supervision I was going to have the perfect wig. A wig pact was sealed between us, uneven and loving explorers of new worlds.

One afternoon Linda and I converged on the wig shop. Leon and his assistants welcomed us warmly. We got our cups of coffee and set out to examine the possible wigs for me. I was fatigued and sad. I could feel the professional care of Leon and Linda's tender compassion. I could also perceive that Leon and Linda had already made a secret pact to do a good job for me and not let me get away with any nonsense. I could see that those two meant business, wig business.

Leon got one wig after another, discussing color, thickness of hair, shape, fitting. Linda moved around me like a lioness around her cub, fiercely staring at each hair that stuck out of line. Leon and Linda behaved like two playful but very serious fencers, moving around me, each making a different hand movement to bring out a shape, a hair "touch" to illustrate their point of view about how I should look. Every so often they paused and withdrew a little to let me contemplate my wigged self. We pondered how much underlying gray hair the wig should have, as much as I have, or more, or less. We found ourselves animatedly counting my white hairs. "I have two white hairs and eight brown ones. That is the proportion," I said. "You have a little more," Leon said. "Three out of ten." Linda frowned, "Four out of ten?" Leon and I jumped in unison, "That is too much." We were caught in the passion of counting hairs, and, noticing it, we all three laughed. We returned to the method of trial and error.

Finally a wig emerged, not the same one as on the previous visit, but an improved version of it that prompted Leon to step back to contemplate the effect and brought Linda to stop circling after three of four turns around me. I was transfixed, my eyes glued to my image on the mirror. Like a small child who recognizes itself for the first time in a reflected image, I laughed with pleasure as though I had found a "me" I thought I had lost. It was a simple, magic moment of silent consensus. Linda unglued me from the mirror by exclaiming excitedly, "Aunt, it is great. It is *really* great!" Leon smiled down on me from his observing distance with the complacent expression of the professional man who knew that the magic moment was coming.

We all three talked excitedly, making remarks about little improvements here and there. Our voices sounded like the voices of children who have just got a new toy. We played around a few more minutes.

Leon was in no hurry. He seemed to know that we, the bold ones, needed time to settle down and find peace in our newly wigged condition.

After a while he said that he wanted me to comb my hair exactly as I wanted it, or, if I preferred, he would do it. I laughed and said I was going to show him how my hair, *my own hair*, shaped its own lovely wavy tricks. I asked for a spray bottle with water and, recalling my mother's actions and my aunt's amazement, I repeated once more the simple trick of getting my curls to fall into place, making it look as though I had just come out of the hairdresser. Leon, like my aunts long ago, showed proper admiration for my hair's tricks. Then he produced a Polaroid camera and asked me to stand against a white background set up specially for taking photographs. He took several pictures of me from various angles. Then he called Terry, his assistant, the person who was to tailor the wig for me. She came in, measuring tape in hand, and, like an anthropologist, proceeded to measure my head at different levels. The pictures were made, the measurements taken, the customers were satisfied, and the deal was sealed. It was time to pay the two-thirds down of a handsome amount of money, $450. Leon quickly said that my health insurance would reimburse me because the wig was part of my treatment. When the wig was ready, he would give me the papers and receipts to submit to the insurer. I was to obtain a prescription for a wig from my oncologist. I laughed in my medical heart. I thought that only doll doctors prescribed hair for maltreated toys. Now I learned that "real" doctors prescribe real wigs for real bald dolls. I felt a kind of kinship with dolls I had seen in repair shops, dolls that had suffered from the love of their owners.

Terry, the assistant, said she would call me when the wig was ready. I would to be taught how to put it on and how to comb it, and then I would have a final, detailed fitting of each strand of hair. Linda and I left, partners in hair matters, agreeing to go together again for the final fitting. We had dinner in a small restaurant. Inevitably we ended up talking about the young men who besieged or disregarded her available heart, and we spoke about the predicaments of a young and accomplished maiden in the eternally bewildering labyrinth of love between men and women.

I was to get my first dose of chemotherapy. Knowing how sick I could get, I had planned to get the wig a few days in advance so as to minimize my troubles.

Eight days after we had found the "me wig," Terry called to say that
I could come in and take the wig with me after learning how to put it
on. We arranged for a day mutually convenient for the three of us,
Terry, Linda, and me.

The day came mantled in a heavy snowfall. The radio announced
that everything was closing. The main roads were being kept open by
constant clearing. Terry called and asked me to come as early as
possible. I had no way to contact Linda. We agreed that I would go, we
would do all the work, and I would wait until Linda came so as not to
let her be stranded. Once I got there, we decided to try the wig on to
see if Linda could tell whether or not I was wearing a wig. Terry and I
found a pleasurable complicity in this idea.

It took a little more than an hour to go over every detail. Terry and
I started the process of personal knowledge. I learned that she was
Irish, had been orphaned at birth and brought up by nuns in an
orphanage, had been rescued in adolescence by some relatives, and
later had been brought to the U.S.A., and married to a sadistic man.
(Her father was an alcoholic who could not care for her and her
siblings.) Her husband began to drink. Finally she divorced him. Now
in her late forties, she was engaged to marry a good man. She had
moved here to live with him before marriage so as not to repeat her
earlier mistake. She had no children. She had not wanted them.
"Children," she said knowingly, "suffer too much in this world." She
spoke of her pain softly, in a matter-of-fact way, with the sober
distance of those who have known true despair and have made peace
with their lot.

I felt gratitude. She had shared a life of sorrows with me in a few
narrative moments. Now we could say "we" because we were both
"acquainted with grief." I told her my sorrows as simply as I could. I
mean my past sorrows of physical pain, of feeling alone, and of the
other strifes of life. I told her of my father's prolonged illness when I
was a child and of the social isolation of the family as a result. I
revealed the story of a broken engagement in my early twenties and of
the great struggle to get my degree against the will of my family and
without financial aid. I told her of an abdominal condition that had
required multiple surgery when I was in my late 20s. A delicate and
unimposing intimacy warmed us in the small space of the mirrored
parlor where she, the orphaned child-woman, was helping me, the
scared child-woman, with my pain of today.

Linda came and began her lioness round, exclaiming, "I can't believe it! You can't tell. It is great. You fooled me." Then we all three giggled like school girls sharing a prank. Terry put the wig in a big red box where one of the hated styrofoam white heads was waiting to wear "my" wig. I remembered my hatred of them, those styrofoam heads, and I was surprised that instead of surrendering the hair to me, the head was willing to come with me as my ghostly alter ego in a box. My marveling was interrupted by Terry, who handed me a red plastic bag with the store gifts to me: a red comb, a white and red brush, a box of bobby pins, a strap that went under my chin to hold the wig while I was combing it, and, finally, a bottle of shampoo. I was dutifully grateful and proceeded to pay the remaining portion of my bill.

I let myself be convinced to buy a gray turban to cover my head while at home, where I was unwilling to wear the wig.

Linda and I left the shop together. She was holding the red box tightly, like a great treasure. The wig episode being over, I was now to go willingly to the slaughterhouse to get my first cocktail of lethal chemotherapy. I had to offer my hair to the killers. I could not help thinking, when I held the wig in my hand for the first time, that I was like the Indians of the Amazon River holding the hair of their murdered enemies in their victorious hands. The difference in this case was that I was both the victor warrior and the victim trophy.

4

Chemotherapy

I had to report now to Dr. Nagle for the final scrutiny to see if he found me fit for chemotherapy. Dr. Nagle, blood reports in hand, extended a friendly hand and invited me into the office. We talked about my having recovered quite well from surgery in the course of four weeks. All the lab reports, he informed me, were normal, and all we needed to do was to decide on the date of the first chemotherapy. I said that I was ready and eager to start right away, not because I wanted it but because my eyes were fixed on the date it would be over. He repeated that I needed eight treatments, spaced every three weeks if my white count, platelets, and other indicators of my body tolerance of the chemicals suggested that it was safe to keep to the schedule as planned.

I told him that I responded very poorly to antiemetics and that it was my explicit request that none be give to me. I had already found Coke syrup, the old medication for vomiting, in a pharmacy, and I was determined to fight vomiting and nausea on my own. I also told him that I had had a long chat with a very learned Chinese doctor, a practitioner of ancient oriental herbal medicine, and that he had shown me publications indicating that Chinese patients under the same treatment with chemotherapy seemed to benefit from specially prescribed herbal medicines to increase white cells, diminish nausea and vomiting, and protect the gastrointestinal tract. Some of the medicines, he added, also could help with the fatigue that plagues the patients on chemotherapy. Dr. Nagle listened attentively and inquired if the Chinese doctor, Dr. Chang, had the drugs available. I answered that he did and showed him the publications Dr. Chang had given me. He said that anything that could help me was welcome. He said that I should try the herbal medicines if I felt comfortable with them. I said that I did. When one is afraid of pain, illness, and death, 3,000 years of painstaking Chinese observations are not to be disregarded by a proud Westerner about to take brutally destructive drugs. I felt relieved and a bit proud, like a special child who is the center of attention, imagining very different medical traditions: ancient Chinese medicine, with her oblique, reflective eyes, and young modern medicine (chemotherapy) not yet (in this field) 50 years old, embracing me in their universal care.

Then, trembling, I asked myself and Dr. Nagle about my prognosis. I knew I was trying to deceive myself. I knew statistics are not people. I knew the doctor could not say anything about *me*. But still, in the mood of the special child I wanted to hear something, a statistical fairy tale to hold on to in moments of great fright. All I wanted, I think, was a little room to maneuver, a sidewalk of hope to totter along during the dark winter of chemotherapy.

I knew when the doctor spoke that he was balancing on the tightrope between truth and uncertainty, meaningful hope and despair. His voice had the soft, well-pondered pitch of those who prophesy unwillingly. He selected his words one by one, like a poet, to give his voice a consoling cadence. "You probably," he said, "will be free of metastases for five or ten years. Nobody knows."

"Well," I said, as frightened as I was relieved, and appealing to the wellspring of sad humor still in me, "I am not yet taking the trip to eternity."

"The *train* to eternity," he said reflectively [I had thought of an airplane], "stops at many stations." I smiled gratefully and looked into his eyes, knowing he had learned the art of saying the right words at the right time.

He got up quietly and said he was going to call Monique, who was to be my personal nurse through the treatment.

March 8

Monique Paterson, my oncology nurse, came in and began to explain our future meetings for chemotherapy sessions. We agreed on a mutually convenient time and checked all the simple practicalities.

"Can I drive back?" I asked, forgetting that she had told me I could at the time of our first meeting.

"Yes, the effects begin four hours after the injection."

"Can I eat if I am not vomiting?"

"Yes, anything you want."

"What if I have difficulty parking my car?"

"I will give you a special sticker, and they will have a place for you at the garage."

Monique repeated that she was going to be my nurse for the course of the treatments and that she was going to keep a good eye on me. I liked her words. They made me feel that I, a frightened child, had been assigned a nanny to watch over me and to reassure me when I was sure that the spooks in the closet, in the closet of my body, were ready to get me.

This was our second meeting. Monique was pleasant looking, thin, with slightly angular features. Her features reminded me of some of the housewives and seamstresses of the Dutch 17th-century painters. Her face had a certain luminescence, a certain exaltation of otherwise ordinary features. She seemed a bit shy, but poised. That was as much as I knew about her. When looking at her a second time, I felt a feeling of affection and attachment toward her, my assigned companion in my experiences of fear and actual danger. I smiled to myself. I had a wish to hold her hand and have her reassuringly press mine. The worst was over. She gave me the parking sticker, and I promised to be there on Friday at 1:00 P.M.

Now I had to plan for the eventuality that my wishes not to get sick, nauseated and vomiting, would not come true. While driving I thought that if such things did happen (I was determined not to let them happen), I would humor them out and not let a few idiotic bodily reflexes get at me. Me, I concluded once more, had to remain the respected lady of my household. So it occurred to me that I could make comedy out of tragedy. Good friends of my childhood joined in to help out: Charlie Chaplin with his ridiculous outfit, and Stan Laurel and Oliver Hardy with their absurd ideas. I felt that their manner of handling life's miseries with their seriously comical naiveté was the only approach that could make tolerable a whole day of vomiting one's guts out. They, after all, always emerged out of their amazing troubles in one piece!

Amusingly, life joined me in making my comedy more real than planned. Five blocks from my home there is a store that supplies every contraption, artifact, limb, or pad that a sick person may need. The store is small, and with its awkward and startling displays it looks like a minuscule factory for fabricating men and women out of assorted pieces.

The woman who runs it – I had met her before – is always bewildered among her wares and can never remember where things are or how much they cost. She has very large hazel eyes that scan her many shelves in hopeless despair. Usually after a while she asks her computer to tell her where the item is. Not infrequently she has forgotten to place a piece of information in the machine, and not finding an answer in the computer, her now wild eyes begin scanning the shelves all over again.

That afternoon I met with this bewildered owner of human parts and helping contraptions to discuss a practical solution to the problem I had posed to her. "I have in my house," I said, "a woman in her 60s who is having chemotherapy and is vomiting a lot. What do you have to make the whole thing less messy?" She looked at me slowly and carefully. She was empty headed and bewildered but not a fool. She knew I was talking about myself but joined ambiguously in the make believe. "I get you something," she said. Then she began running back and forth frantically because she could not find what she wished to sell me. "What is it?" I asked. "Maybe I can help you find it." "You need a bib," she said. "They made them just for that." Charlie Chaplin, Stan Laurel, and Oliver Hardy all clapped hands together with me. "Please," I said most seriously, "give me the biggest one you have, no matter how big, so we can protect her whole bed." "I have a huge one," she said, "but I can't find it." I inquired about what the box looked like, where it could be, and other identifying details. She told me, with the resigned, fatigued voice of the one who faces a thankless job.

So now we were both running along the shelves. We found little bibs, middle-size bibs, and plastic bibs, but not the "real bibs" made of real white towel to cover the whole bed required by my comedian friends. "I've found them," I said with determination when I discovered that they were in a tight bunch at the level of my feet. They had been there all along. She marveled at the discovery while together we opened the package, and I tried one on. It was perfect. I could tie the clerical looking collar with velcro in the back and let the white rimmed towel float all around me to my feet, hanging from my shoulders, making me a remarkable combination of a high priestess in her holy robes and the best of Molière's patients. I was elated in the midst of my sadness. Now I dashed to select a container for my vomit, one equally efficient and ridiculous. A gigantic yellow plastic basin for $1.29 seemed the perfect match. Round as it was and bright yellow, seated now on top of the white mega-bib, it gave the impression of an immense egg.

The items selected, it was time to pay. The woman had been pounding frenetically at her computer. Finally she said in despair, "I don't have the price of the bibs. I can't let you take it." "Bill me," I said, "I'll give you my address." "No, no," she said, "I call the factory." She could not get the factory. Then she looked into a book. There was nothing in it about gigantic bib prices. Finally she said, "It is not much. Please take them and next time you come here you pay me." She seemed to fear that I was going to vomit right there. "Well," I said, "that is very generous of you. Let's give it a final trial." I looked at the package, where the price was neatly printed. She dashed to look at it, ran to the cash register, and with a great sigh of relief took my money and packed my gigantic bib and my yellow basin.

My mood had improved beyond recognition. The best of my sense of humor had found in real life an unexpected enactment capable of making a perfect scenario for the comical side of life's tragedies. Carrying my contraptions for vomiting, I felt proudly in the company of Molière and the movie comics. Once at home I rehearsed my act, wearing the bib and playing *Le Malade Imaginaire*. I cut a pretty impressive figure in the mirror.

The woman in the mirror now reminded me of what I did not want to see. The comedy was an act of magic, of exorcism, of word imagery. The image in the mirror would have to remain there like an imaginary movie. "*I*, I will not have nausea. I *will not vomit. I* will not be sick." Like a four year old, I kicked on the floor and hit a pillow with my fists. "I won't. I won't. I won't," I said while still wearing the mega-bib and looking at the basin on the night table. That was my first temper tantrum. I was to have many in the days to come.

March 14

The scenario was ready. Two days after my temper tantrum I was to report for the first treatment. We had agreed that Friday was best for me. I had the whole weekend to rest and recover, and then I could go on with my work and my life. "Go on" was a manner of speaking used to exorcise evil events that could take over my life. I had been properly informed by Monique that many complications might be added to the simple nausea and vomiting: skin rashes, blisters and sores in my mouth, a drastic lowering of my blood count, diarrhea, neurological complications, and, maybe later, leukemia. "Some patients," she said, painfully reciting an obligatory litany to those sentenced to chemotherapy, "have to be hospitalized."

While Monique was saying these things, a defying poor devil awoke inside me and talked in counterpoint with her while jumping up and down indignantly on her feet. "Out with it: no skin rash. Out with it: no mouth sores. Out with it: no hospitalization. No, no, and NO!!!" The devil's little horns pointed at Monique to attack her if any of her prophecies of doom came to pass.

The poor devil in me was brave and courageous that day when Monique was telling me what might happen. But now that I was parking my car in the hospital garage and trying to rehearse the fateful words to the receptionist, "I am here for chemotherapy," the poor devil was nowhere to be found. I was afraid, as afraid as prisoners must be when they are taken to unknown buildings where terrible tortures will be inflicted on them. I walked slowly, searching for the green hospital card in my pocketbook. I cleared my throat to be able to have a full voice and to veil the whimpering voice of fear.

The receptionist, a young, exuberantly made up woman, asked with the voice of a person forced to ask boring questions, "Where are you going?"

"To chemotherapy," I said in the lowest of voices because I was ashamed and did not want anybody to overhear me.

"Do you have a green card?" she asked.

"Yes," I said, and I gave it to her with the same inhibited disposition. She looked at her desk and picked out the blue sheet for chemotherapy from a shelf with many slots for assorted forms. I understood immediately that carrying that form in my hand was an explicit announcement of my trip to chemoland. She stamped the form and gave it to me together with my card. I rolled the form over and tried to make it invisible while I went up in the elevator.

At the nurses' station the routine repeated itself, but the scenario was different. There, sitting or standing, going in and out of different offices, were my wigged fellow chemoland inhabitants. They did not seem to notice that by reporting to the oncology receptionist the "abracadabra" words, "I am here for chemotherapy," I was entering their private world. I had a secret and fearful wish that at least one of them would come to me and shake my hand and say, "Welcome. Do not be afraid. See! We have been here some time. You'll get used to it." I felt, while waiting for a few minutes, a great need to make eye contact with one of them, with any of them. I couldn't. Those who had somebody with them were talking or sitting quietly. Others seemed too sick to do anything but be sick. The rest seemed to be doing their living in an inner universe, on the other side of their pupils, which were glassy, like muddy water.

I noticed that I was sitting on the edge of my chair. Self-consciously, I sat back, hoping nobody had observed my uneasiness. I could see that I was developing a psychiatric syndrome, a chemotherapy persecution paranoia, as though the whole universe were spying on me and whispering that I was having this terrible "thing" called "cancer treatment." My self-diagnosis brought me to my better senses, and I laughed faintly – that was as much as I could laugh – at my capacity to transform my fears into persecution. I could not finish my reflections. Monique came, sat next to me with a genuine smile, and, looking into my eyes (I was so grateful), said, "Are you ready? If you are, we can go now." I nodded and followed her like a lamb to the slaughter house.

The slaughter house was very pleasant. It had eight cubicles separated by sliding cloth curtains in such a way that patients could elect to be alone or remain in view of the other patients. It also had a horizontal S-shaped couch like the ones at the Red Cross for blood donors, a little table, a TV set, and in the wall all the paraphernalia for medical emergencies. Monique invited me to make myself comfortable on the couch. It did not take any effort to follow her suggestion. The couch took my body into its curvy surface and made me feel held and relaxed.

Monique sat next to me and explained what she was going to do. First, she would get a saline I.V. going to get enough fluids in my system (before coming I had to drink four glasses of water) to protect my bladder from the concentration of chemicals so potent that they could damage the lining of the bladder. Then she was going to inject the three drugs into the I.V. tube, one after the other.

Monique skillfully started the I.V. and chatted about a few more things and gave me some necessary warnings. I would not feel anything until four hours after the "chemo." I could eat anything I wanted and drink a little wine as usual with my dinner. I could feel very nauseated with my dinner. I could feel very nauseated and vomit a lot. I interrupted her and said firmly, "Monique, I won't have any of that. I told you, I won't have any of that. (I couldn't help laughing, observing a professional women in her 50s talking with the imperiousness of the Queen in Alice's Wonderland.) *I have thrown a temper tantrum* and *I have said I won't have any of that.*" We both laughed at my outburst, but I felt the need to add, "Don't you laugh. It will work." We laughed again.

Then we talked about her because we were becoming friends for the journey. She told me how her pregnancy was going, and her face lit up. The baby was not yet kicking, but she had been examined and all was well. It was her first child and the first grandchild for her husband's family. The baby was due late in July, which meant she would be on maternity leave at the time of my last two treatments. I felt sad and a bit scared because I had already began to cling to her with the hope and determination with which a victim of shipwreck hangs on to a faithfully floating piece of wood.

We talked about names for the baby, and the baby's sex and clothes and other matters. We felt a womanly camaraderie, a tenderness about this new life growing in her womb. I reflected privately about the words of Mircea Eliade: "In all mythologies life and death form a complementary cycle." Aware as I was of receiving, just at that moment, a deadly drug to kill my very killer cancer, I found in those words a certain philosophical resignation, a mild awareness of belonging to a broader universe of things being born and dying.

Monique said that I had enough saline in my system and that now she was going to give me the drugs. First was Cytoxan. It came in a small I.V. bottle prepared by the pharmacist for my treatment. They had calculated my body surface and measured the drug accordingly. After the Cytoxan came an injection of amber yellow Methotrexate, and, finally, another injection of 5-fluoruracil. The three together make the acronym CMF In my best mischievous moments I read those letters as Certified Medical Ferociousness. I kept the reading secret, as spies keep decoded words. When the yellow Methotrexate entered my veins, it was soon followed by a tingling metallic sensation on the upper part of my nose and in the back of my mouth. I told that to Monique. She looked at me at once and said, "You are very sensitive. Most people feel it only later, and usually they feel it as a sinus congestion. You may feel that and some mild bone ache in the next 24 hours." She gave me the last one: 5-fluoruracil, and the whole thing was over.

Altogether it took an hour and a half. Monique asked me to stay on the couch for a few more minutes. Suddenly a smiling black woman, who identified herself as Patsy, came in with a cart full of cookies and beverages. She asked me what I wanted. I felt entitled to indulge myself fully. I asked for cookies and chocolate. They were delicious, more delicious than I had imagined. I was aware that their enhanced flavor was not due to their quality but to their meaning: the living act of eating. And, so, my first "chemo" was over. I put on my coat, said good-bye, and walked to my car repeating my exorcising words: "I won't have nausea. I won't vomit." Entering my home, I had the feeling of recognition and strangeness one experiences after having gone abroad for several weeks.

March 22

[This entry continues the narrative of the previous day.] The middle of the afternoon was sunny and soft and mild. I did not feel anything special upon arrival at my house. According to Monique I still had two to three hours before any symptoms appeared. This time of the afternoon is a time when I walk in the neighborhood either for pleasure or to run some errands. "Life has to go on as usual," I said to myself, put my coat back on, and went out. I met some friends and neighbors who knew of my "chemo" and who wondered what I was doing on the street just after my first treatment. I said that I was doing what I always did, walking a little around the neighborhood to keep my joints oiled and enjoying the sunny afternoon. They pondered my wisdom and warned me to be careful. I smiled, half grateful, half indignant. I wanted this caring. I feared my impediment, my being a visible indicator of my own fragility. We parted. I walked under a cloud of dark thoughts that followed me, encircling my head like bees humming around the bee hive. The fear of their stinging power gripped me. My legs felt as if they were made of cotton, but they did not bend under their weight because I myself had become fluffy and weightless and a bit unreal. A bird appeared from nowhere – it was not supposed to be there so early in the season. The little creature chirped a few unexpected sounds and then flew away. The bird, small and ordinary in its feathery brown coat, had accomplished what an orchestra could not have done at that moment: it had delivered a message of unconcerned life, of the simple joy of being there, alone, out of season, chirping while perched on a barren branch. Gratitude rushed from my heart to my lips and I said to the now absent bird, "Thank you for celebrating your little life." I was feeling the smallness of my own life.

The gospel words came to mind, "See the lilies of the valley and the birds in the fields. My Father in heaven takes care of them." I knew that the quotation was not accurate, but they were certainly sufficient to evoke a feeling of being part of a universe that is properly cared for by a Father who looks after the little ones.

I kept on walking. The buzzing bees of my dark thoughts had left me. The softness of the afternoon wrapped me in its faint luminescence. A delicate calm, made of invisible threads of many remembered smiles and bygone tender afternoons, settled on me as I watched the soothing predictability of the sun setting for the day.

I returned home to find my phone ringing every five minutes. All my friends wanted to be with me, to offer something, to know how I was feeling. In a few minutes Linda came to be with me that first night. We had a quiet dinner with a bit of wine, chatted about immaterial subjects, and went to bed early. We were both aware that the awful things that were supposed to happen were not happening. I had no nausea, no need to vomit. My facial bones, particularly around the sinuses, were a bit sore and had a congested feeling. My legs ached a little. That was all. We went to bed. The night was uneventful, but sleep was fitful. I was asleep, but in some strange way I had never experienced before, not exactly asleep. My mind kept on flashing endless, disconnected images, like the irregular shapes of a kaleidoscope, shapes incapable of forming a geometrically harmonious design. Three or four times during the night I was awakened by hot flashes. I had begun to have them a couple of months earlier. They were the result of the sudden withdrawal of estrogen and progesterone that I had been taking prior to the discovery of the cancer.

The perspiration and the hot flashes seemed to be increased by the chemotherapy. Later I was to learn that the drugs themselves added to the disturbances of peripheral blood circulation caused by the pituitary gland's efforts to stimulate the production of sex hormones. The efforts were all in the brain because the body had no responsive organ capable of releasing any quantity of sex hormones.

I had already been introduced to this symptom when I stopped all hormones the day after Dr. Marcus called me about the pathologist's report. I was already used to countless nights of waking up in a sea of perspiration, hot as a worker in a foundry, red faced and suffocating. It did not take me long to realize at the beginning of the early episodes that I was facing a most unpleasant and protracted symptom for which there is no other treatment than the hormones I could not take anymore. Once more I was called to the humbling act of accepting limitations and impotence in facing this internal change of weather, from intense hot and wet skin, to moments of feeling very cold and incapable of warming up without an electric blanket. I remembered a description of the Sahara Desert I had made in my adolescence: the sun burns the naked surface of the sand during the day, and by night the chill of darkness fractures the rocks, inflexible to such extremes of temperature change. I have always loved the solitary majesty of deserts. The night of my first chemotherapy I felt a familiar solidarity with the burning sands, the chilly nights, the hallucinatory images that meet the solitary walker of a vast desert.

Morning came, and I awoke to a mild feeling of nausea. I vigorously repeated my exorcism: "I won't vomit. I won't be sick." The bottle of coke syrup was waiting for me. I drank my first teaspoonful and hurried to have breakfast – a light breakfast – because Linda was still asleep, and it was too early to wake her up. After breakfast I still had a slight queasiness. I took another teaspoon of Coke syrup with the incantation: "I won't vomit. I won't be sick." I had perfected the rhythm, tone, and pitch of recitation. I said it aloud for all evil spirits to hear it. It had now acquired a certain ridiculous majesty of power and domination, a convincing *ex opere operato* sort of esoteric, sacramental, exorcising force. It did seem to have force, a force I did not feel. I was exhausted, a bit disoriented, although in a mild fog. It seemed to be a neurological effect of some of the drugs. I went back to

bed and dozed on and off, waiting for Linda to get up. 1
was like that, a bit unreal. I was in a body that felt differ
way it had felt before. It is not easy to describe. I was nc
sick. But I had a feeling of ill being, of being beaten down
left without energy. It evoked in me a languid and sad mood of
resignation and abandonment, a wish to give in to powers that I did
not control.

So the day went by, and Sunday came as an undifferentiated
continuation of Saturday. The problem with Sunday was that it was
inexorably followed by Monday, and on Monday I had to get up at
6:00 A.M. and begin my work at 7:00. I did not want to work. I did not
want to see anybody. I did not want to have to come out of my languid
and melancholic mood. I did not want to demand that my body
function like a normal social body when I felt so changed internally. I
needed an act of will to force my body. I only wanted to rest and
withdraw. I had to make it do all it had done before. It was in this way,
by the need to work and to appear normal myself, that for the first
time in my life I became the puppeteer of my own body, and that
happened on the Monday after my first chemotherapy.

March 29

My friend Robin called from Durham, North Carolina, to see how I
was doing. She had had breast cancer three years earlier and had gone
through the same process and treatment. She had kept it a secret, and
it was upon the revelation of my own cancer that she told me about
herself. She spoke with the knowing and respectful compassion of
those who have gone through an ordeal. We compared notes about
our experiences. She too had waited for nausea and vomiting, feeling
that she was missing something that had to come but that did not
come. She described how she had felt a bit cheated and disappointed
even while she was relieved. We both mentioned that not having the
symptoms was like not paying for the cure, a sort of breaking a secret
law of health prices that said that one had to suffer to get well, as
though having cancer were the result of some unmentioned sin, some
unrecognized wickedness that demanded sacrificial offerings.

We laughed sadly, observing that the cancer was like a nodal point,
the center of a spider web attracting to itself the guilt of forgotten

childhood deeds and "evil" thoughts. We acknowledged that there was in her, while she was undergoing her treatment, and in me now, a need to attend to those deadly threads of the spider's web, to be able to keep a clear mind about having cancer and chemotherapy, to escape the added and unnecessary suffering of self-chastisement and self-accusation. We recalled Susan Sontag's book in which she defends herself vigorously against some superficial conclusion of ongoing research about personality traits and breast cancer. Some people seemed pleased to conclude that the victim of breast cancer has done it to herself by being a sad and depressed character. We noticed once more that in facing the thread of death, magic is called to duty to prevent the killer cancer from harming unsuspecting victims who do not carry the dispelling amulet. Those who seem to say "You got cancer *because* you were always depressed" appear to console themselves by holding tightly to the hopeful formula, "If I am not depressed, I won't get it."

Robin mentioned that she no longer had any use for her bald head cap and some cookbooks for a better diet that she had collected to help herself. She said she was going to mail it all to me. We laughed, saying that cancer had made us like sisters or a kind of twins. I said I would feel like her wearing her cap. She said she had several, but there was one that she preferred and that would be the best for me. She was going to send that one to me.

Robin is a kind and intelligent person whose respectfulness one can count on. She made me feel that I was not alone in this journey of life and death. She had descended to the Hades of chemotherapy and had returned to her normal life. Her presence, her modulation of past excruciating feelings, her message that the treatment does come to an end, gave me hope that the six-month journey would one day come to an end and I too would be free of symptoms for some years or perhaps—I was afraid to hope—for life.

Her package arrived on a Friday afternoon. It contained a patterned brown and yellow cap, a booklet from the American Cancer Society explaining chemotherapy and its effects, and a cookbook with nutritious recipes for cancer patients. I tried on the cap to rehearse for my future baldness. It looked nice enough on me even though no one could hide baldness by wearing it. It was strange enough on a head like mine to advertise its cover-up purpose. Then, just for the fun of it, I tied it under my chin rather than on the back of my head. I could not repress the laughter in seeing my image in the mirror. I looked like a Colonial New England woman, quaintly Puritanical. That evening Carmen and Gregory came for dinner, and I told them how I lookd with the cap on. Carmen began to laugh just hearing the way I phrased it. Her laughter was uncontrollable when I put the cap on, tied under my chin. She had no choice but to agree. I did look like a woman "of the colonies." The phrase was to become a shared expression.

Now everything was ready: wig, cap, medication, and the practical arrangements of getting someone to help out with cooking and food. I had a cleaning person who kept my house in order and did the food-shopping for me. Now, however, in my weakened condition I needed help with cooking and doing all the small household chores. I discovered that the so-called small chores—watering plants, feeding the cat, sewing on a button, picking up a pair of shoes from the shoemaker, and preparing ordinary simple food—took an hour and a half each day. I had not realized it while I was doing these things as a matter of course when I was in good health. As I mentioned earlier, finding a person to help out proved to be quite an enterprise. I called six agencies, all of which advertised every possible kind of help one could imagine. All of them said in their advertisements that you should not worry if you became sick because they were there. Well, they only seemed to be there, at least for me. The first agency sent a woman who would work only eight hours a day. She came once for three hours to pacify the agency and me because no one else could be found. Finally the agency manager confessed that she could get no one. The next agency, after endless calls, had the manager yelling at me, saying that she had no one. The third agency sent a woman who came for two days, promised to work for me for the six months I needed her, and then disappeared into nowhere at the end of the second day after telling me that her "aunt in New York" was gravely ill, even though she could not name either the hospital her aunt was in or the illness that had made her ill.

The next woman, a polite and attractive looking black woman from the Caribbean, proved to be blatantly psychotic. It took her half an hour to put on the uniform of sorts that she carried with her. A few minutes later I found an unknown man in the living room. He had rung the bell trying to sell something, and she had invited him in as if he were an old friend. Fortunately, he was a real salesman. I had not yet recovered from that shock when I smelled the pungent odor of gas. I ran to the kitchen to find it smelling intensely of gas, the jet open without a flame and the woman about to light a match. I screamed just in time to stop her. I opened all the windows, even though the temperature outside was 20° F. The woman seemed oblivious to the danger and continued smiling pleasantly as she asked me what to do next. Luckily, it was close to the time for her to leave. I paid her and sat there supervising the last few things she had to do. After this experience I continued to tell my friends that I needed someone to help and asked them to be on the lookout for a good woman.

I called some other agencies. Finally an agency provided a woman who seemed capable of cooking a few things under guidance and of replacing me in my chores. Watching this pleasant and eager woman I realized the precariousness of her situation. Like the others, she had just arrived in town from New York and was living with a cousin and her 14-year-old son. Her precariousness was also my precariousness. She could disappear as fast as she had appeared.

Meanwhile, one of my friends had located another woman helper, a woman with a home and a husband, she too was an illegal alien from the Caribbean. I tried her out, and she committed herself to work for me. So I had to dismiss – not without sadness, knowing that I was her only source of income – my pleasant looking black woman. It was unfortunate that my limitations now collided with her precariousness because she seemed to me like some one who justly deserved to have a job to support herself. I said so when I called her, explaining that I no longer needed her help. She was gracious and resigned, and we both felt sad to sever our budding relationship of two weeks. Once more some misquoted gospel text came to me: "Those who have should have even more." She had nothing.

Now I had to learn to have help at a level I had not been used to, to create a system that would work automatically, to spare my energies. So I created a personal cookbook where I wrote my invented recipes and indexed the ones I had obtained from some other sources. I had fun doing it, putting into written words things I had done all my life without thinking. I developed a small feeling of pride in "kitchen mastery." My next book was a book of orders and things to be done in a question and answer format. Mary, my household helper, could write her questions and I would solve her problems in writing after she had gone. The system began to work, and I felt that one more weight had been lifted from my shoulders.

Meanwhile all my friends, in their sad impotence to do anything to change my condition, found that feeding me was a way of shared consolation. So they came one after the other with their gifts of fish, bacon and beans, full meals ready to go into the microwave, fruits, candy, cookies, crackers and cheese. My freezer and my pantry were bursting with all varieties of delicious food. So it was that each meal became either a pleasant act of mastery (to teach Mary) or a friendly incorporation of a gift of love. "Love," I said to one of my friends, "has the marvelous advantage of having no calories."

April 6

Mastery of my new circumstances brought to my life a certain routine and ritual. Some of my energies required a prescribed order of things with do's and don'ts. Do's were the things that *I* had to do: see my patients, answer my correspondence, teach my university course, take care of my physical being, make sure I did not isolate myself, and bring myself to all my doctors' appointments.

The don'ts were anything I could get someone else to do for me: take a taxi if I had a heavy day instead of driving myself, and get someone to pick up video tapes or books from the library for me or prescriptions from the pharmacy.

Interesting things began to happen. I discovered a side of the world I had not yet known: the hidden organization of many services for those who are housebound or very restricted, as I was. I found that I could get any medication delivered directly to my door if I paid $2.00 extra. I could organize errands and call a person who, for a moderate fee, would have them done for me. I could strike a contract with a taxi company, get a coupon book from them, and have them automatically come to my place to pick me up at fixed times for fixed appointments. I neither needed cash nor had to haggle over anything. The rate was fixed, based on miles, and all I had to do was to sign the coupon and give it to the driver. I found out that some people cook at their home or yours. Some of them prepare gourmet meals ready to go in the microwave and deliver them into your freezer, miraculously finding room for them in a full freezer.

These discoveries awoke complex feelings in me. The first was relief at having found an invisible network of helpers I could use if I needed to. The joy was not free from the sad awareness that all this was possible for me to have because I could afford it, although it clearly overburdened my budget. Nonetheless I did have the money to pay for it. I thought about the women bewildered about having lost a breast who are poor. They may have several children and an equally bewildered husband with whom they are not able to speak about the maiming of their bodies and the threat of death. I could see these women withdrawing into their fright and carrying the burden of their emotional pain and the weight of their duties as forced laborers, not unlike oar-paddling slaves of ancient times chained to their seats, repeating mechanically, under the angry eye of a slave master, the endless gestures of their duties. I had known a woman like those slaves. Thinking at the time that "she had cancer" and she could not cope with it, I had not reflected compassionately about her helpless fright and submission. I had dismissed her because I did not belong to the world of those who "have cancer." Today, in my heart, I felt a wish that I could have talked with her, that I had had the awareness and wisdom to understand what was happening to her.

I stood now a bit tall and proud of having organized the three-ring circus of my life, which used to be busy but simple. Taxis came and went. Delivery people left their merchandise in my hands. Friends unloaded their love-food. My regular household helper cleaned and shopped as usual. Mary, my new helper, cooked my recipes and mastered the art of leaving meals ready to go into the microwave. One day my mind went back to a childhood storybook. I did not remember the whole story, but an illustration in the book. There was—I saw the page in my mind—a small circus ring and hoops in it for lions to go through, stools for elephants to stand on one leg, a huge motorcycle for a monkey to ride on, and a very fat woman dressed in a furiously red bathing suit, her legs apart, showing her amazing fat collection. Finally, in the center of the ring was a very tall ringmaster with striped black pants and an enormously bursting chest covered by a starched white shirt, crowned by a small black tie and coated with a long, double-tailed gala jacket. The man had a fine long moustache standing upward at its ends and a monocle in his left eye. His right hand held an enormous whip, while his left hand was extended and open, showing how he, a true gentleman of the ring, mastered beasts and men with a simple gesture of his greatly puffed up person. Such a display of grandeur in a little circus had a very comical effect. I knew – and I smiled in learning it – that I was like that man: all puffed up because I too kept my little circus going. Neither the ringmaster nor I – in our shared puffiness – looked at all at the helpers who were attending to every detail of the performance, humbly keeping the act together.

April 12

My efforts to master the little circus – my new medical life of appointments and tests, my fatigue, and my previous life of work, teaching, and friends – left little time for thoughts that demanded attention but were constantly dismissed in favor of their more practical and pushy competitors. Those were thoughts about the future, life and death, life with cancer, death from cancer. Dreadful visions passed through my mind. They had an overtone of horror and helplessness like Hieronymus Bosch's paintings. I began to look at snatches of my mind's paintings of the future made by the unknown artist awakened by the depth of my fright. I saw myself pale, with white hair, skeletonlike, eyes sunken and staring from their depth with sad despair. It took courage to look at that dilapidated woman whom my mind insisted on calling "me." I did not want her to be me, but she looked at me with moist eyes, begging, hoping I'd recognize her and accept her as "*me*." Every fiber in me said, "No!" Every fiber in me knew that she could be "me" tomorrow. An unspeakable wish to disown her clashed with my moral determination to face myself and my cancer at every level of my being.

I forced myself to look at that *myself* that the artist of my depths – more honest and more dramatic than I – had placed in front of my mind's eye. I saw first the woman's hands. They were bony, wasted, frail, holding to the rail of a hospital bed with the gesture of a child holding mother's hand in a moment of worry. She was wearing a blue-dotted hospital gown, opening in the back. It was not properly tied, so it fell open on one side, uncovering a bit of her right shoulder and a bit of an old mastectomy scar. My eye could ascend the road of her skinny arms, where wasted muscles offered a cord under thin skin for the eye to go up to the sunken shape and the protruding collar bones of the upper chest. The eye now found two diverging cords going from the center of the lower neck to the right and the left sides of the jaw bone, stretching out the edges of her wrinkled face. The angles of her jaw led the eye to the ears, beautiful once upon a time but now too large for that diminished figure. The eyes converged on her nose. It suffered from the same disproportion. It had once been harmonious with that face, but now its bony structure, unmodulated by the lost flesh, was one more sign of the devastation, the dilapidation of being that was eroding the woman and her face.

Suddenly my eyes met her eyes. At that moment I recognized that the "me" I was seeing in my mind had come from a moment in my past. I had met that woman 25 years before. We met for approximately 30 seconds. Those 30 seconds held the ponderousness of an entire life, the tragedy of unavoidable recognition, of insoluble tragedy. The entirety of the drama came to the moist surface of the woman's hazel eyes when our eyes met. They were kind, maternal, pleading eyes, asking me with the urgency of despair a question I could not answer. The intensity of the interrogation pierced my entire being, moved me to tears, which for her sake I tried to contain. In my despair, not knowing better, I put my hand on hers holding a nursing home bed rail. I looked deeply into her eyes, until the gentleness of our human encounter and silent communication replaced the hopeless terror veiling her pupils. I smiled as tenderly as I could—a prescription I had not learned in medical school. I felt her hand releasing the tension under my hand. I said softly, "Bye now," and left, feeling her gaze fixed on the back of my head like an invisible line of unworded serenity over uncontrollable fear.

Here is the story of my encounter with the woman whose name I never knew, whose silent dialogue with me was limited to those 30 seconds. I was covering ambulance calls in Metropolitan Washington, and it was my unlucky assignment to go every morning to a huge, state-owned nursing home to sign the death certificates for those who had died in their sleep and who had to remain in their beds until a doctor could check their cold bodies, certify they were dead, and write the death certificate based on whatever medical information was at hand. The beds where the corpses were lying were in an enormous room with double rows of beds. When the dead person was in a bed at the end of the corridor of beds, I, wearing my white intern's uniform and carrying my black doctor's bag, would walk toward the dead person. The terrified eyes of all those who had not died during the night followed me as though they could control their own death by watching me. The question, formulated or unformulated, in their imploring looks was "When are you coming for me?" I felt each time like the angel of death, the announcer of the end, the fatal marker of the last moment of a life I had not met but who could not leave this world without my signature.

The images of their terrified, imploring faces returned to me now like Old Testament prophets' visions of doom and destruction. There was a sort of perverse mockery in the way they returned to me, a sort of Talion law of revengeful retribution: "Now it is your turn. Now you'll be waiting for nurses and doctors to come while your fellow cancerous companions die one after the other, and you'll never know when you'll be plucked out from the world of the living."

My mind returned to the reality of what I had seen in the waiting room of the oncology clinic. The patients there did not look dilapidated and abandoned, as the patients in the nursing home had. Their middle-class money had covered up with wigs, props, plastic surgery and make up the defects of their mutilated, wasted bodies. Under the pleasantness of their poised dignity, however, it was possible to see the advances cancer had made in their bodies. Every so often, someone would come in a wheel chair or on a stretcher, carried in hurriedly by ambulance. Those were called "unexpected patients," that is, those who were supposed to keep going but whose body had given a new signal of infirmity: bleeding, pneumonia, pain, obstruction of organs, or some other of the mechanical failures of the human machinery.

I watched "them" while attempting to use the pronoun "we" to name myself among "them." My semantic watcher refused to use "we." Fear, sheer, ordinary fear, warned me to use the magical denier, to use the pronouns as amulets and to hold tightly to the "I," as though by saying "them" and "I," I could segregate myself and my cancer away from their curse and bad luck.

My imagination, also inspired by fear and an uncertain future, did not believe in verbal magical tricks and much to my despair kept placing *me*, an older, white haired, thinner, paler, sadder looking *me*, in the old state-owned nursing home. There I lay imprisoned by the metal bars of my safety bed, waiting and waiting in idle despair for a death that I feared as much as I might need it to liberate me from my desolation.

I was learning my lesson: fear is an emotion to be respected, taken seriously, attended to with kindness and an open heart. Facing fear, we are all children of nature, creatures subject to pain and death, two unavoidable realities beyond the limits of the intellect. I sensed that such a fear could be alleviated only by the tender concern and holding that adults provide to a child when the child, feeling small, threatened, and overpowered by the creatures of his reality and of his fantasy, needs to cry within the protecting cradle of the parental lap.

Tears of fear, cried softly with a listening friend who *would not* try to console but simply let the fear be, have the effect of a summer storm. At first all is bleak and threatening and the world seems about to come to an end. The thunder and lightening and rain appear to confirm that the end has come. Then, when the sky has finished its cosmic crying and has returned unexpectedly to its original blue, the earth, dressed in a misty veil and perfumed with all the scents of newly bathed stones and plants, acquires a radiant new serenity, crowned by the chirping celebration of the summer birds.

There is an unnamed tenderness that develops among people who have been together through a storm of tears. As with nature, the aftermath brings a new serenity, a way of accepting one's pain and fear and of knowing that one is accepted when one is fearful and pained.

April 19

I have not talked much about the plastic surgery and the plastic surgeon. The surgeon was a distinguished looking gentleman, very easy going. He was always willing to give broad latitude to any decision that had to be made. His voice had a particular inflection, a sort of trademark of his way of practicing his specialty. His sentences started in a low key, a slow and well-tempered tone that went on, progressively increasing its pitch, though very slightly, until it made something like a somersault at the end, a pirouette suggesting playfulness and hope. That manner of speaking and his extremely relaxed demeanor conveyed a sense of "nothing tremendous is going on in here" and a certain elation about what had to be done.

One day, still during the initial consultation, when I was saying that his procedures as a plastic surgeon reminded me of my playing at being a doctor with my sister at age six or seven, he broke into frank laughter and said, with noticeable complacency, "I never grew beyond five. I used to make mud pies, and I loved it. I can still play, now as a surgeon, as I did then. It was, and it is, a lot of fun."

I loved him for his words. He was a very reputable expert whose success had neither intoxicated him nor suffocated the child who provides the joy of playing with our adult professional sublimations. I loved him also because I could bring with me my playfulness and my fear, knowing that a man who still plays like a five-year-old knows how a five-year-old can dissolve into tears a second after laughing with pleasure. I had started off on the right foot with him, so I looked forward to seeing him as a child looks forward to recess and playing with a favorite playmate.

As I said, immediately after the mastectomy, the surgeon, Dr. Robbins, left the operating room, and Dr. Keily continued the operation, placing under my pectoral muscle something called the expander. The contraption is an ordinary plastic bag, round and flat, that ends in a tube at the bottom. The tube is six centimeters long and is called the port because it is used to inject saline solution into the bag, week by week, until through the bag's expansion, the skin of the chest expands to the size of the remaining breast. When the expansion reaches that size, the bag is removed and a permanent implant in the shape of an ordinary breast is placed under the muscle and skin. Dr. Keily explained to me that this method was invented by a young plastic surgeon who watched the skin of his wife's abdomen expand and stretch with her pregnant uterus. It occurred to him that what the skin of the abdomen could do naturally, the skin of the chest after surgical mastectomy could do under the pressure of a progressively expanding bag, a simple reasoning whose transformation into a surgical contraption has brought relief to many maimed women.

I was now the beneficiary of an observant husband and father to be, and Dr. Keily, in turn, could play doctor to his heart's content by injecting 50 cc of saline solution biweekly into the port of my expander.

April 26

The progressively expanding bag introduced some problems to the task of keeping my breast "looking" normal under my clothes. I had to find a brassiere that would accommodate the changes, one that would permit me to remove some padding each time the expander grew a bit bigger. This practical and pedestrian matter, even one so important for my self-image and social ease, brought my good five-year-old plastic surgeon to a moment of confusion. He seemed a bit embarrassed to talk about such matters. His voice lost the final somersault and trailed off to a slowed-down mumbling about "many companies" and "certain people" who know about these matters. He had no nurse during those early weeks, so there was no one to resort to. I had the feeling that the five-year-old child who played with bags and mud pies did not want to be found looking at and handling his mother's underwear in the bedroom chest.

No one had addressed this problem with me before. Neither my surgeon nor the nurses in the oncology unit had considered the simple fact that I couldn't go out displaying a one-breasted chest. No one seemed to be willing to talk about anything beyond my skin, as though my life ended at my anatomical boundary. While I was in the hospital, any questions about clothes and brassieres were answered with, "We'll talk about that later." Finally, when the discharge date was set and everybody behaved as though I could go out naked, I went to the nurses' station and in no meek terms demanded that the head nurse find me a person, a phone number, or something else to provide me with the necessary help. She shuffled the pages of a black book she had in her desk, called a mysterious number, and told me that before the day was over a "very reliable woman" would come to help me out.

The day went by hour after hour without any sign of the "reliable woman." I was becoming increasingly angry and frustrated because I knew that once I was home it would be by far more difficult to solve the problem. It was the eighth day after my surgery, and I was well enough to walk back and forth in the surgical unit's corridors. At 9:50 P.M., when I was going back to my room to get into bed, a woman dressed in a mink coat and perched on very high heels dashed in the direction of my room. The night nurse whom I had been pestering to keep calling the woman's shop shouted with relief, "There she is!" The woman introduced herself as Elizabeth, shook hands with me in the solemn manner usually reserved for someone serving a death sentence, and proceeded to talk very quickly about her services. She was perhaps 60 years old, had straw-colored, dyed blonde hair and the eyes of a missionary among black Africans. They conveyed, in their sad, pale blue indifference, the fatigue of a savior who feels the burden of her yoke and perceives the futility of her efforts. She did not talk directly to me. She delivered her credo with responsible punctuation of the main points to make sure that the message was properly presented even if she did not care to prepare my ears to welcome the gospel of postmastectomy resurrection. It became obvious to me that she too had had cancer and that this mission of hers at 10:00 P.M., after she had been running all day preaching her little sermon, was her way of mastering the same pain I had, the pain of being maimed.

She told me her company could help me with anything related to my mastectomy, gave me her card, and said, in her pained, hurried, "believe me please" voice, that I did not have to be ashamed of having lost my breast. To console me, she produced from her bag a little rose made of enameled metal that was supposed to be a symbol for celebrating the femaleness still left in me. I love roses of any kind, but I instantly hated that one. It felt to me like an absurd amulet of the secret society of one-breasted women, who wanted to make believe that you can console yourself with trinkets. I contained my anger because the woman seemed more burdened with her pain than I was with mine. She could not make contact with me as a person and continued to produce more items from her bag.

The next one was a piece of silken material, a bag of an oval shape, the size of the cup of my brassiere. She double checked my bra size and asked me for my bra. Then she showed me how to proceed. The silken bag had an opening in the back. The woman now produced a cotton-looking stuffing that she called "acrylic wool." She explained that it was better than cotton because use did not flatten it out as happens with cotton. She stuffed the little bag until it had the size of what had been my right breast. Then, with a solemn admonition, she instructed me to pin it in *from the outside* part of the bra with three safety pins to make sure I would not pierce my skin if the pin opened accidentally. She insisted I should do as she said. I promised to obey. She asked me whether I had any more questions. I didn't. The contraption was simple enough, and the poor woman seemed driven to finish her job and dash out to continue her "acrylic wool" breasting mission. She did not look at me but hurried to place everything back into her little bag. Finally with the expression of someone who has fulfilled a burdensome duty, she wished me well and left, stooped over her sad burdens and her high heels.

She helped me more than she could have imagined. I had enough distance from the absurd cheap enamel rose and the comical "acrylic breast" to know that meaning in life and the preservation of identity after mastectomy had to go beyond these gimmicks. It had to include the acceptance of paradoxical justice, where illness and pain are not signs and symbols of punishment and persecution. It had to integrate an internal system of justice that did not violate the needs of the factors involved: the society of human beings, the victim of cancer, and the cancerous process itself.

That mink-wrapped woman, Elizabeth, coming with her gifts in the late hours of the night taught me a lesson: if I was to live meaningfully, I could not sugar coat what had happened to me. I had to face it squarely and call each anatomical change, each emotion, each social difficulty by its proper name and truly face the magnitude of the changes that had come upon me. I must have meant what I said to myself that night because I lost the rose, and no matter how carefully I searched for it, I have not been able to find it.

The whole experience of stuffing a brassiere to simulate a breast left me bewildered by the lack of emotional help for women with mastectomies. I was able to do what I did because all my friends, male and female, who came to my room could talk directly and even with some humor about the sad fact that I had to use some contraption of sorts to look normal. I am sure from what I managed to learn from the nurses that I was, in that respect, the exception among mastectomized women.

I felt very sorry for those who had no one to talk to them and very angry with my profession, the medical profession, for its inability to deal with our bodies as the living bodies of social persons.

May 3

My chemotherapy was now well underway. Every three weeks on Friday I was to report at 1:00 P.M. to my nurse for the I.V. infusion of the three anticancer drugs that were supposed to wipe out all malignant cells from my body. Each time it felt as though I was willingly going to poison myself, perhaps not unlike medieval and renaissance kings who took small amounts of poison each day to be able to survive the heavy doses maliciously dropped by enemies into their wine cups.

The procedure had now become a routine composed of a few steps. First, my blood had to be checked to make sure I had enough red cells, white cells, and platelets. Then the oncologist had to check that I was well and free of symptoms, particularly free of any infection. This was essential because the drugs deeply affected my immune system, and after each injection my biological defenses were depleted, like an army that has lost half of its troops to the plague sent secretly by the enemy. When the tests revealed that there were enough troops – white cells – to weather the oncoming massacre, the decision to get the next treatment was confirmed and I got my CMF.

My life was becoming a patterned, three-week routine, a gruesome menstrual cycle of changes without ovulation of any sort, a menstrual cycle where not just one egg lost the chance to become a human life but where all new cells of my body were aborted in their very moment of conception, a menstrual cycle centered on the Herodian massacre of innocents with the expressed intention of killing the unwanted one in the mass murder.

To know that *my* body was the field of a war I could not control gave me a painfully acute feeling of impotence, of being foreign to my own flesh and bones. My poor body, so truly mine at one level, was at another a foreign territory, a wasteland of life and death capable of controlling my very living or dying. The wasteland could concede me the right to germinate, bloom, and complete my allotted life cycle, or it could clamp down on my existence and let the wild multipliers, the cells of doom, the invaders of all private territories suffocate my life.

The awareness of the almost incomprehensible relation to my body filled me with as many contradictory feelings as I am capable of having: love for a body I knew so well and on whose fabric I had embedded every loved person I had met in my journey, their love in my flesh, my life in my flesh. That was my body. Their betrayals, the caresses they did not give, the kisses I did not give, the bodies I did not embrace, that was my body too. This body of love, of betrayal, and of human intercourse was mine, totally, completely mine. More than that, that body was *me* and my personal itinerary. Now I had to face this other, cancerous, body within my body, with rules and regulations of its own, not caring that its wild actions were performed on *me* and could finally, if uncontrolled, kill me.

A deep, impotent anger rose from the depth of my human pride, resenting from the core the independence of my body from *me*. I hated being its serf now that it could become my executioner. I mistrusted the same body I joyfully had taken for granted in health, when it was so delightfully nimble and so naturally at the service of my fancies. It was no longer at the service of my fancies. The fatigue caused by the chemotherapy was intense and persistent. The first week after the infusion of the drugs I was in a fog, had trouble concentrating, always was a bit nauseated and had a constant feeling of dizziness and of general malaise. Each task that I had naturally carried out before, almost without awareness, now required a conscious, willful effort. The second week after each injection the fatigue abated a little, but then some abdominal cramps, diarrhea, and skin rashes, as well as corneal irritation that made my eyes watery all the time, made the lessening of the fatigue only a displacement of miseries from one part of my body to another.

The third week after the injections was always better and almost free of symptoms with the exception of some remaining disturbance of appetite, body temperature regulation, and some sleep disturbance. The improvement evoked a glimmer of hope each time, a return of memories of the days when I was in command of my body. The hope was short lived because the third week had arrived, and now it was I who took my poor body, my friend and helper, to the slaughterhouse. All its renewed cells were to be killed like unaware innocent children in the hope of killing the special one, the powerful one, that could dethrone *me* and kill me.

So it went, week after week: a dance of life and death, of desolation and hope, of impotence and mastery between my body and myself. In the course of time, urged on by the intensity of the experience and the complexity of my feelings, I entered slowly into the land of serene humility. I can only talk about it in broad religious terms. It was an acceptance of not owning my life or any life. I felt that I was a creature, that is, a being created by somebody or something else, that my life, my body, my awareness were all things that I simultaneously owned and did not own at all. They were given to me without my consent and did not need me for me to have them. Out of this awareness I developed a kinship with all existing things. We all share the same paradox of being: we exist yet do not own our being, our own existence. I felt humbled, brought down from my human pride to a simple fellowship with "all things great and small."

Now that I had gone through my battle with the angel of the Lord in my night of fear, I, like Jacob, came out a bit maimed (he limped afterwards); but after I had looked at my Maker face to face, my body, like Jacob's, could show in its defectiveness that I had found my measure as a creature.

It was at this point of wrestling with myself and the Maker of us all that I remembered a beloved forgotten friend, the joyous Francis of Assisi and *The Canticle of Brother Sun* in which he calls all other creatures his sisters and brothers. I ran to read the canticle again and found comfort in saying with him, "Brother Sun, Sister Water." While my lips named all living things as "brother" and "sister," I felt the consolation of participating in a larger universe of life and death, a universe that encompassed and surrounded my frightened little life.

May 3, Late Evening

I have not talked much about family and friends. Like so many Americans, children of immigrants to this land of hope, my extended family was in another land, far away, reachable only by letter or telephone. My immediate family was dispersed all over the country, miles away. I was alone in my hour of tribulation, alone like so many other American women of my age, in sole charge of my universe and my responsibilities.

No one could leave his or her own universe to come and be with me. Children cannot be neglected; jobs cannot be ignored. Each one of us is enclosed in a particular universe of connections, and we cannot leave it to attend to a woman who has breast cancer. Such is the nature of our individualistic society where the extended family has broken up into small groups of three or four members, nuclear families that more frequently than not leave an older woman, her maternal task fulfilled long ago, alone with her interests and her friends. In that respect I was one of the many American women who live alone and who are accountable only to themselves.

In such circumstances, friends become as precious as air, as water, as a restful bed.

The cursed word cancer, the name of a flesh-devouring vice, runs from mouth to mouth like a herald of death, awakening in each friendly heart a long-forgotten call to combat. Each friend responds to the call as ordinary citizens do when called to arms to defend the nation. No one knows what kind of soldier will come forth when his name is called. Some are brave, and some are cowards. Some would prefer to carry the wounded. Some will be heroes because of their very effort to overcome their fear, and some will run AWOL as soon as the sergeant turns his vigilant eye from them.

My friends showed in their responses to the herald's call the varieties of friendly experience in facing a friend accompanied by the monster cancer. Gregory sobbed on the other side of the telephone line, saying in between tears, "Oh, no! Oh, no! Not you, Madeleine! No!" His tears were as warm and tender as mother's milk. We both cried, taking turns at consoling each other. His desolation consoled me. I knew I could share despair and bitter sorrow with him. Alexander and Martha dropped their voices a few decibels and then called forth a fierce determination to kill the monster and save me. They were splendidly efficient. In a few hours they had called every consultant I might want to see. They put their heads together like a think tank to survey the territory of my needs and wants and made lists of everything, including the thoughts I could have and the ones I could not. In short, they acclaimed themselves generals in my war. They would watch over me. They would act respectfully and firmly on my behalf. They were also very tender. I still felt moved by the gift of the Indian purse they had been saving for my birthday. In their wish to console me they gave me the gift as an "anticipation." I could feel that the gift carried impotent affection that could show their love but was unable to cure. I was grateful for their love and for their gift.

Wila, who was acquainted with sorrow, having lost a child to a terrible illness, responded with calm, kind words and offered to do anything I wanted. She was infantry, a foot soldier, taking orders with faithful and simple devotion. It was she who came with me to the hospital on a horrible stormy night two weeks after the surgery when I found that I was getting an infection in the surgical wound. It was she who thought about very simple details of everyday life to make my life more bearable. I knew that I could ask her for the most idiotic favor, and she would carry out my wish without roaring with laughter at my extravagance. I knew I could laugh with her and be silly and crazy, and she would remain a level-headed friend.

Rachel, who like Wila was divorced and living alone, responded with a solemn voice and a deep sigh. She spoke slowly, carefully, with beautiful words of concern. She sat down, as a matter of course, for a

dialogue. For her, friendship is a dialogue, deep, honest, soul searching, her compassion is expressed in undistorted truth. So we sat,
without tears, and with sober and tender voices pondered the depth of
my plight and marveled at the fragility of our human life. I knew that
I could entrust her with the most unthinkable thoughts of my
torments and my efforts to make sense of terribly frightening worries.

Larry and Robin had faced illness in their families, terrible illness.
They responded with great anguish and anger on my behalf. They felt
anger that I, their friend, had been wounded by the ultimate fiend.
Larry moved around the room like a man ready to kill the devil itself.
He said, "Damn!" with every other word along with some other words
not fit to print. He warned me not to think I was going to die. In a fit
of impassioned eloquence, he made a lofty speech about "those fools
on the street who do not know they can die just now" while he was
trying to get me to understand that the only difference between them
and me was that I knew I "could die." He worked himself up into a
most excited state while deep, large tears were rolling down his cheeks
and mine. Robin cried quietly, a faithful witness to true sorrow. I knew
that I could pour out every fear I had, tears and all, in their presence,
and that we would all three have a most needed crying session.

Bernard and Jill came as soon as I called. They came in a hurry,
bringing candy, said a few perfunctory words, and, before I had the
time to appraise what was going on, left. They were two soldiers who
went AWOL. I did not see them at all after that visit. They never called.

Joe and Blondie, my good friends of many, many years were there,
simply *there* all the time. They were friends during good and bad
weather. They brought me a sober and self-possessed joy, a distancing
sobriety, that made room for sorrow and good cheer when the little
steps of recovery came along. They were like fairies: they appeared
from nowhere whenever I needed them.

My friends from other parts of the country and from abroad called
as soon as a mutual friend told them. The phone carried their many
voices through uncountable miles of telephone wires bringing concern, consolation, good wishes, good cheer, in a moving symphony of
human love.

I must be one of the luckiest of human beings because in my darkest
hour my friends encircled me with their care, their honest reactions,
their faithful services, their dialogues, their prayers, and even a few
well meant childish pranks to make me laugh. These and many others

were my friends. Most of them were faithful, a few were very afraid, and a couple were really gone from my life.

Next there were colleagues and acquaintances. Some avoided me as though I carried the pest in my breath. Others claimed they did not want to disturb me, although I knew they did not want to find themselves disturbed. Others played hot and cold, not knowing *how* to talk with me. Others felt it their duty to keep me well fed. They came to visit me laden with gifts. Some came with words and food. Some dashed to the kitchen, dropped their packages, and left with light hands and heavy hearts.

There is no gain in having cancer. There is no gain in being frightened to death. There is, however, a paradoxical joy, a joy that words cannot describe, in finding the love of friends at one's bedside. Such love makes us immortal in the truest sense. Not even death can kill that unnamed event that happens among friends. So it was that in my most sorrowful hours, in the night of my human terror, I found myself revived beyond my quivering flesh by the tender breath of friendly love.

The pain of the few who betrayed me can not compare with the affection of those who stayed with me. Those who had to run away because of their fear of me did not know that they were the losers. They lost the opportunity to discover one of the deepest moments of friendship. That was their loss. For my part, I felt sad and betrayed, angry and ashamed. Each emotion had its own source. The sadness came from the knowledge that I had lost a friend I thought I had. The betrayal tapped on the feelings I had entrusted to the friendship, the confidences I had made, the private thoughts and feelings I had shared while believing that there was a mutuality of feeling. The anger piggybacked on the betrayal. Those friends who had run from the common bond had robbed me of my trust, of my good faith in what I had thought we had shared together. All three feelings – sadness, betrayal, and anger – were colored by shame. In spite of my clarity of thought, a small, persistent voice kept on whispering in my ear that it was my fault. They had abandoned me, the voice insisted, because I was not good enough for them, or because I was stupid enough to believe that social conveniences were true friendships. It was, I knew, the shame of being rejected just at the moment when one has readied oneself to be kissed, the shame of being seen wanting.

May 10

I had been told that more likely than not I would lose my hair. I was at this point in the sixth treatment, and of the eight I was to receive, as I said jokingly, I still had "my mop on the top." Monique smiled sadly and said that even with the last treatment I could lose my hair. Dr. Nagle, more optimistic, said vigorously, with the gesture of a boy throwing a ball, "Good! Get the damn wig, and throw it out, and forget about it." I smiled at the time because I knew that I did not have the courage to "forget about it" while the possibility of becoming bald still existed.

Doctor and nurse had warned me to watch out carefully for any bleeding, however small. They told me I could feel confused, be short of breath, and have more difficulty with my balance. They had insisted that if I had any fever or chills, I was to call them at once, at home if necessary. The doctor had given me three numbers where I could reach him at any time.

They had added that I could have skin rashes and corneal irritation. Finally they had said with solemn voices that I was going to feel very fatigued for the entire period and there was nothing to do about it but to live with it.

Everybody had told me repeatedly that I should be frank, *selfish*, and *bold* in requesting that my needs be attended to. I very much liked the "order" that I should be selfish and laughed a bit when I heard it, not knowing then how much I was going to need it, particularly to handle the fatigue.

Monique told me about a symptom called "anticipatory nausea and vomiting." Proud as I am, I told myself that I was not going to become a Pavlovian dog. I was not going to surrender to the anticipatory anxiety about receiving the treatments and the expectation of being sick afterwards. I said to myself and to Monique that I was determined not to vomit even when I knew I could not prevent the nausea. As I have said, I had decided to develop a simple method, that is, to throw a sort of tantrum, kicking on the floor when the nausea came and saying aloud, like a two year old, "No! No! and No! I won't vomit."

It was my good luck that the method worked well for four treatments. After the fifth, however, I woke up at 5:30 in the morning the Saturday after the Friday treatment violently nauseated and with my mouth full of a very acid liquid, so that I had no choice but to vomit. I was still practically asleep, standing in the bathroom vomiting. There was no time for my tantrum. Then, after I recovered my composure for a few seconds, I was awake enough to recall my techniques and ways of fighting nausea before it became a vicious circle of vomiting and more nausea.

I grabbed the little bottle of Coke syrup (the original formula of the good old pharmacist, John Pember, who in 1886 created what was to become the world-famous Coca Cola) and drank a teaspoon while practicing deep breathing exercises to control the diaphragmatic contractions started by the vomiting. This fifth time had become an unequal battle. My body seemed possessed by the nausea, and I was like a sea captain trying to control his vessel in a storm while strong waves rocked it. It took 45 minutes of my standing there breathing, drinking the Coke syrup, and literally kicking on the floor and hitting the bathroom basin with my fist, saying, "No, I will not vomit! No!" until the diaphragm gave up its sea waves.

I was left with a strong nausea and a sensitivity to smells and even to fast movements, to the point that I had to slow down for 48 hours until it subsided.

Perhaps·what brought the nausea on was my previous condition. I had been sick with the flu for over five weeks, and I had a deep cough with a lot of mucus coming up. First I had the flu with a temperature of 102° and great prostration. It improved enough for me to get my fifth treatment. A few days later, I got a cold, first a head cold, then a sore throat, and finally chest congestion and a dry cough that progressed to a deep, cavernous cough. I was at the tail end of that episode when I went for my sixth treatment. Now it was too late. Once more I was overcome by the nausea. It subsided after 48 hours, but I was left with stomach queasiness, some abdominal cramps, and a mild gastric distress for many days. Even on the Friday before the chemotherapy I had a sense of gastric malaise.

The day before the treatment I had a surprising experience. I *thought* about the treatment, and, suddenly, a wave of nausea came over me. I recalled at once Monique's words about "anticipatory nausea and vomiting." Much to my regret I *was* becoming a "Pavlovian dog." The vomiting that Saturday morning after the fifth treatment did it. Perhaps my pride was hurt because I had lost control of my body.

Perhaps my reflexes—my Pavlovian reflexes—had made a neural connection without conscious consent. Be that as it may, I was in the grip of a conditioned reflex. The thought of the treatment, the visualization in my mind of the saline solution bag, the bottle of Cytoxan, and the syringe with the yellow Methotrexate and the other syringe with the 5-fluoruracile instantaneously evoked in me an intense nausea. I realized that unless I could interfere with the Pavlovian signals, interrupting the connections between them and my nausea, I was going to be in trouble for the next two months for the seventh and eighth treatments and for the future should they ever be necessary.

I could not, however, do anything about this sixth injection. I woke up a 2:00 A.M. with my mouth full of vomit. This time I vomited my entire dinner as though I had just eaten it. My stomach had kept it untouched for seven hours. I could not stop vomiting for several minutes. I was even nauseated at the thought of taking a teaspoon of Coke syrup. The spell subsided, and I returned to bed for an hour or so, when I was again awaked—my mouth full of watery saliva, and the diaphragmatic waves. A terribly acidic liquid came out of me with full force. Again I fought to control it but to no avail. I seemed to be filled to the brim with the acid stuff, and I had no choice but to vomit it. I went back to bed again only to be awakened in the same manner, the episode repeating itself three or four more times throughout the night.

In the morning I was exhausted, my throat hurt, and my spirits were lower than ever. Every so often the memory of the injection returned with another wave of nausea.

It was now *a fact*. I had become a Pavlovian dog, literally salivating a watery saliva and feeling diaphragmatic contractions each time I saw in my mind the medications in the treatment situation. I felt terribly discouraged. I had been taken over by the symptoms in spite of all my brave determination. The events that were taking place in my body were bigger than *me*. In my low spirits, made into a coward by my impotence, I realized that I had to take seriously my situation as a "conditioned dog." I had to "decondition" myself if I was to have a livable life during the next few months. My manual from the National Cancer Institute, a branch of the U. S. Department of Health and Human Services, recommended relaxation techniques and deep-breathing exercises as well as thinking that the drug is for one's benefit. They also recommended the use of imagery and of tension-relaxing techniques. I carefully read their advice because it had become obvious to me that I needed help immediately if I was to control a symptom that could very soon control me.

May 24

I realized that one cannot trick the body. I could not blindly apply the suggestions of the National Cancer Institute booklet. The words written there had to circulate through me, mind and body, and become a deeply felt conviction, a wish, and finally an act of will, carrying out a series of sequential psychic processes, images, thoughts, commands and physical actions.

I questioned myself about *how* to convince a body and a mind, repelled and nauseated by destructive, almost lethal drugs, that they were for my own good.

The first discovery jumped to my mind with vicious force. I felt a true *hatred* for the drugs. All of me, each cell, each organ, each member, raised a clamoring shout of rebellion. Images of dying cells, poisoned all at once in every organ of my body, flashed before my mind's eye. All of me cried, "Stop it! Stop it! Don't murder my body! Stop it."

I found myself saying in my mind, "I hate these treatments. I hate them." A darting thought tempted, "You can stop the chemotherapy. Quit. Quit now. You have had enough."

Hearing my inner screaming horrified me. I had not realized that beneath my brave defiance and courageous conscious efforts subterranean murky waters of rejection and hatred had been gathering force and had now overcome the dam of my conscious containment. The ancient fight between conscious and unconscious wishes was now raging within me, compressing me between their contradictory forces and intents.

The hour was critical. Humility, simplicity of heart, and cleverness were all called forth in this hour of confrontation with myself. I had to humbly admit that I had in fact become a Pavlovian dog. I had to accept the sorrowful yelping of that frightened, beaten dog in me. The soft voice of Dr. James Herriot, the English veterinarian and author, came to me to talk tenderly to "all things great and small" trembling in my frightened body. "You have the right to howl," I said to the death-sentenced cells who (I thought of them as little Lilliputian people) had innocently started their first and only adolescent sexual blooming. "You will be killed," I continued, "for having dared to blossom and reproduce. Cry because the spring of your life will be your tomb." I watched them in my mind's eye. I felt their "pain." My chemotherapy, I thought, was a war, intended, as all wars are said to be intended, to sacrifice the part—the young lives—for the whole of the nation, for the whole of the body. That is what chemotherapy is: a war, a massive, atomic bomblike blast to the enemy, the inner traitorous cells, whose wild, youthful power of multiplication could invade every corner of my bodily territory, accomplishing with their triumphant life, my death.

The image of their uncontainable advance on the territory of "me" raised in me an urgency for defensive measures. I surprised myself by awakening to a belligerent mood. Now a war cry arose in my mind, "Kill them. Stop them. Do not let them kill you," and, as the imagery books had suggested (I learned I was more suggestible than I had thought), I "saw" the drugs entering the cancer cells, those cells wild with reproductive urgency, and saw the drugs shrinking them to nothing. I fantasized that their rotting debris would make me sick. The realist in me, like a commanding general looking at the battlefield, saw that the corpses were intermingled: those of the cells that gave me life, maimed in their healthy youth, and those of the monstrous cancer cells that brought *me* the tidings of death. Looking sadly at so much destruction, I said soberly, "This war, this chemical battlefield is for you. They must die if you are to live. These deaths are the price of your life." I noticed, saying these words, that a certain conviction, a feeling of righteous war, a crusade of salvation, was rising within me like the sun dawning after a long winter night.

I felt now that any imagery I used to decondition the Pavlovian dog in me would not be a gimmick, a trick for survival, but a tool in the service of a renewed wish to keep my life.

Humbled by the complexity of my mental processes, I felt ready to submit to the suggestions of the manual of the National Cancer Institute:

> Some patients suffer nausea and vomiting just at the thought of having their drug treatments. The problem (known as "anticipatory nausea and vomiting") results from anxiety about receiving the treatments and

the expectation of being sick afterwards. There are a number of methods you can use to cope with the stresses of cancer and its treatment.

Reading the sentence carefully made me realize that to decondition myself I had to find exactly what evoked the reflex. A survey of my experience revealed two different sources of the nausea. One was the image of the syringe with the yellow Methotraxate and the metallic smell and taste in my nostrils and mouth that followed almost instantly after I received the injection. The other image was that simply inhaling, at that moment of remembering the immediate effect of the injection, made my body reproduce the sensations in my nose and mouth as though I were receiving the injection at that very moment. Nausea followed the memory. "You must undo this negative association and create a positive one," said the Pavlov in me.

The manual suggested thinking that the yellow substance was going to cure me. I heeded the suggestion and tried to figure out the best associations to accomplish the goal. The simplest seemed to be the most useful. I reproduced in my mind the same scene, smell, and taste as I experienced during the chemotherapy and said to myself, "This you have to endure to save your life. It is not so bad a disturbance in comparison with what the drugs do *for* you. Bear it patiently. Look, (I imagine looking straight at the syringe with the yellow liquid) it is just a small injection; it will help you. Thank *it* for *its* help." I "talked" to the liquid and thanked it for its power to help me. Then I remembered St. Francis's invitation to bless the Lord for all existing things. I added to St. Francis's long list a blessing for the existence of Methotrexate and other anticancer drugs, saying, "Blessed be the minds of the scientists that discovered these creatures of salvation. Blessed be the power of these molecules to kill my cancer cells. Blessed be those who give them to me. Blessed be the Lord that made these molecules."

The exercise brought a serene feeling to my soul. The harmony of the universe so beautifully celebrated by Saint Francis had now quietly brought some luminous peace to my imagery of death and destruction. Encouraged by the result, I said to myself that I had to repeat these thoughts and feelings many times over until their healing power seeped through the many layers that led in me to the murky subterranean waters of hatred and despair.

I made it a habit similar to morning and evening prayer to repeat those blessings over and over during the day when fear and discouragement threatened to overtake me.

I had started out trying to handle my nausea. I had ended up with healing words for my torn and frightened soul.

May 29

I still had to face the possibility that all this good effort would not work and that in spite of it all I could vomit and be nauseated. I knew I had to appeal to the strongest and most humble part of me, the person in charge of myself, capable of accepting the shortcomings and reverses of life.

I had to ask myself, what if I did vomit and become nauseated and sick for two more months? The very asking of the question seemed to bring some peace of mind as though facing it courageously brought a measure of contentment, of acceptance. My thoughts moved slowly as I pondered the question. I realized the depth of my fears. I was truly afraid of the power the symptoms had over me, of their capacity to take center stage in my life, as the fatigue already had done. I had learned to live around my fatigue, letting it control what I could and could not do. The possibility of persistent nausea and the abominable metallic sensation in my mouth and nostrils brought back the sensations and the accompanying nausea. I knew at that point that I needed the courage of a coward. I had to go through it, if it had to be, scared, trembling, humiliated, angered that I had no choice. The coward, having accepted that fact, amazed me with its little voice of resigned realism. "Well," it said, "you just go one minute at a time. After all, nausea is nausea, not death." (Good reasoning, I thought.) "Two months," it continued, "seems long, but one way or another the days follow one another, and finally it will be over. You just endure a little nausea here, a little nausea there. It will be the same with the metallic sensations. Close your eyes, and be patient. It is bad, but you have no choice, no escape. So take it, even if you and I (your coward *me*) hate it."

It amazed me to witness this new division of me in dialogue with myself. Accepting that a proud woman like me could be a shivering, irrational, afflicted coward seemed to provide a measure of common sense to help me face what I had to go through.

"Well," I said, "that is it. I am a coward, and *I like it* because it gives me the feeling that cowards have the right to exist." Suddenly I found myself sympathetic, in a new sisterhood with many others: those who faint at the sight of blood, who kick and scream when they need an injection, who cannot face the dark, and who believe that their closets are filled with spooks. I imagined joining hands with these scared fellow human beings in a gesture of alliance to give us, the cowards, the courage to endure the real and imagined horrors of the world.

Then the other side of me, the thinker, the ringmaster, returned to its former place, ready to invent a plan of action.

Pavlovian reasoning was called forth now. How does one impede the reinforcement of a conditioned reflex? "By impeding the formation of associations between a stimulus and a sensation," said the Pavlovian thinker. "What can I do," I asked, "to achieve such a thing?" It occurred to me that if I could avoid feeling the metallic sensations during the chemotherapy, perhaps the already existing reflex would extinguish itself for lack of reinforcement. A strong smell that blocked the other could do it. I remembered that a friend had sent me a bottle of a delicious, penetrating perfume as a gift. I tried the experiment by placing it in my nostrils and inhaling very deeply. It seemed to be strong enough to take over my sense of smell. I decided to take the bottle to the hospital. I also thought that I had to block my sense of taste, perhaps with something sugary.

Armed with perfume and cookies, I went for my seventh treatment. Monique and I talked about my predicament. She agreed that I could try my Pavlovian system. I noticed that she listened very attentively and was doing her part of the thinking. As soon as she installed the bottle of Cytoxan (which also gives a bit of a metallic taste), I filled up my mouth with cookies, letting them dissolve slowly. Every few minutes I placed perfume on my index finger and inhaled it as deeply as I could. I felt encouraged because it seemed to work. I did not experience any flavor or smell but those of the cookies and the perfume. Monique suggested adding 10 mg. of Decadron to help control the side effects. I accepted her suggestion. When the time came for the Methotrexate, Monique, without saying a word, did her part. She hid the syringe from me so I would not see the yellow liquid while she was injecting it. I was grateful for her thoughtfulness because I had not made plans to undo the association between sight of the syringe with the yellow fluid and the metallic sensation.

So it went: while she was injecting me with a hidden syringe, I was frantically inhaling perfume and chewing cookies all at the same time. It worked! I did not feel the sensations at all and apparently I did not form associations among cookies, perfume, and anticancer drugs.

Monique and I had developed a very congenial relationship. She knew I was writing down my experiences and had asked me to bring them with me to read an excerpt to her. The previous time, though I intended to bring my notebook, I had forgotten it. This time I remembered to take it with me and read to her what I had written last about my hatred of the drugs. She listened attentively while I read to her with the self-consciousness of an elementary school girl reading her English composition to the teacher. After all, Monique was the great expert in these matters of feelings and sensations about chemotherapy. Each day she treated four or five persons with mild or terrible cancers, and she certainly knew the private hells they were going through. I was a bit afraid of seeming banal or melodramatic. Her opinion was at this moment as valuable as that of the *New York Times* critic.

When I finished reading, I cast my eyes down, bashfully, waiting for her comments. To my great relief she said that what I had written was good and that I should publish it. What was good, she said, was that I talked plainly about how deeply I disliked it all, a subject that others who have described the experience seem to gloss over. I asked timidly about the literary aspect of my writing, which concerns me as much as the contents. She said that she felt it was good. I feared she was not a knowledgeable enough critic in such matters, but, needing approval as much as I did, I chose to agree with her and think of myself as an accomplished writer. In a flickering vision I saw my name and the title of the book discussed in the Sunday Book Review section of the *New York Times*. It was a needed pinch of grandiosity! I left the hospital in a good mood, hoping that my final two treatments would not be as distressing as the first six had been.

Once at home, I became aware that I had more energy than when I had left for the hospital. The Decadron (a more potent form of cortisone) was acting on me as a stimulant. That night I did not sleep for a minute, but I was not tired. Happily it was Friday night, and I did not have to worry about working the following day. I did not, however, have the metallic sensations or more than just a bit of nausea, easily assuaged with a few teaspoons here and there of Coke syrup. I felt glad with the trading of symptoms. One can recover easily from a transient episode of insomnia, while being nauseated a good part of the time is a most disagreeable and depressing experience.

My spirits began to lift. I felt that perhaps the next eight weeks of chemotherapy and its side effects would not be so bad. I even permitted myself to imagine that the day would come when I would feel well, like my old energetic self. My imagination could not do the job too well, given the pressing information from all of my body, especially that feeling of being ill, the prostration that follows the first 48 hours after the chemotherapy. The good results of my treatment of the Pavlovian dog brought with them portents of better days to come.

June 7

The long therapeutic process now entered a new phase. I went to see Dr. Robbins, the surgeon, for the second checkup after the surgery. A few minutes later I had the next to last appointment before surgery with the plastic surgeon, Dr. Keily. Both men treated me with great kindness and a buoyant joyfulness that I found very encouraging , particularly because I felt that they meant it for *me*, even if it was their habitual professional stance. When I left their offices I felt that I had two friends willing to help. Such good luck on my part deserved gratitude. Many doctors nowadays do not want any human contact with their patients and are too busy calculating their time and their earnings to see the patient as a person. After my experiences with my two surgeons, I decided to place them on the altar of my patron saints. I saw them both on the same day, one after the other. Their offices are located at the two extremes of a very very long corridor. The secretaries informed each other about my whereabouts because Dr. Robbins was behind schedule. That, too, a secretarial network, gave me a feeling of being in a familiar place where I was somebody, a body whose movements were to be traced from A to B, as teachers of kindergarten children have to do all the time.

Dr. Robbins shook my hand with vigorous enthusiasm and after careful scrutiny declared that I looked very well. I retorted, "Look very well, maybe I do. I just wish I felt as well as you think I look." He then asked about symptoms and side effects. Obviously, I was normally abnormal for my situation, so I passed the test.

Then he examined my breast scars and the mobility of my arm and looked at the work of his colleague, the plastic surgeon, who had been adding saline solution to the implanted expander, making my scar area look like an inflated balloon smaller than the natural left breast. Dr. Robbins was greatly pleased with the evolution of my surgical scar, palpated it, passed his fingers over the area, reading the braille alphabet of flesh communication with fingers capable of reading every dot of the skin. What he read satisfied him. "A beautiful scar," he said, as though he were complimenting my beauty. Pained as I was at having a scar instead of my breast, I still felt that he had done the best he could to help me. I said, "You did a good job." He retorted, "Your scar-tissue formation is excellent." I laughed. We sounded like a mutual admiration society celebrating the jointly accomplished task of leaving me free of cancer for the time being, but maimed there in the right side of my womanly pride.

We talked about what I could and could not do with my right arm. I confessed sheepishly that I had been sawing some wood with a hand saw. He laughed and said I could do anything I wanted. I had full mobility, enough lymph nodes were in place to protect me, and all I had to watch out for were skin infections. He said that the best way to protect myself was to wear gloves while working with materials that could injure my hands even slightly. If I noticed any infection, however small, he said firmly that I was to call him at once.

Dr. Robbins wanted to see me again in six months. He looked at me with the satisfaction of a man who has done a good job, his eyes filled with pride, his well-formed mouth opened, a proud smile supported by a raised chin of uplifted spirits. Watching his shining looks, hearing his words and the mood they expressed, I could not avoid feeling like a minor piece of paradoxical art, a molded chunk of clay that had turned out well. We left wishing each other good luck. His secretary informed me that Dr. Keily's secretary had called to say that he was waiting for me at the other end of the corridor.

I arrived there, and for the first time I did not have to wait 45 minutes to be seen. Dr. Keily was in a reflective mood, as though he were preoccupied with a problem. I fantasized that perhaps one of the patients with severe cancer he had seen for years was very ill or that perhaps he had another concern that kept his mind occupied. He was, as usual, kind and full of comical remarks, even if partially absent. His nurse seemed to share the mood. I felt that they had always been very attentive to me and that I could let them have their preoccupation.

Dr. Keily reviewed my medical record. I asked him how many cc. of saline solution I had in the expander. He said that with the 30 cc he was adding today I had 550 cc. He felt that that was enough. I did not have to return until the next month to see if another few cc would improve the results of the plastic surgery. I also had to come to discuss the final details of the plastic surgery.

As Dr. Robbins had done, Dr. Keily read the braille message written on my breast scar, the skin now expanded under the pressure of the saline-filled balloon. He too felt satisfied and, talking to himself, praised the anatomical development of a small fold under the expander, saying that it was a nice evolution of my skin, which indicated something good for the future. I did not understand much of what he meant, but I did know he was not talking to me but to himself as a surgeon pondering facts and planning strategies.

As I was leaving, I realized that I had grown fond of him and that I had taken my weekly or biweekly visits for granted. I found contact with him uplifting and enjoyable. I found myself thinking that I was going to miss him when the whole thing was over. I asked him how frequently he saw his patients after the surgery. He had said that if there were no complications, I did not need to see him for several weeks, except to arrange for the surgery. The corner of my mind's eye registered a fantasy that I would be part of some research and that he would follow up my case and continue to see me. I smiled at my wishful thinking.

As a physician I know that when we become patients and are treated with kind respect and feel in emotional contact with the doctor, we become grown-up children, wanting the protection of a knowledgeable adult who can console us in our fears and dreads. There is a type of affection one develops for such doctors that differs from any other I know of. It is a mixture of respect and trust, of warm bodily feelings and a bit of playfulness about little things related to the condition that brings one to the doctor's care. It is not unlike some feelings of childhood when all is well with the parents and their bodily ministrations become little games about belly buttons or big toes. While I was walking through the long corridor to leave the hospital my steps were nimble like those of a girl ready to start a game of hopscotch, even though I was still beset by the fatigue of chemotherapy.

June 14

I found, five days before my last treatment, that I had a little more energy than I had had before at the same time of the cycle. Once more I felt a great hatred for the chemicals that made me feel so exhausted, so unable to own my body. I found myself mumbling to the drugs, "I hate you! I hate what you drugs do to me." I did not want to go. I counted several times a day how many more days were left before I had to go. I knew I had no choice if I was at all responsible. Nevertheless, I concocted little plots for escaping, in the manner, I suppose, that people in prison who fear death or torture plan their deliverance.

I forced myself to force myself. I tried to be kind and light handed with my besieged person, and I talked to myself with kind words. So did my friends. Each of them said it in a different way, but all of them said it. "Take courage. It is just one more treatment. Let's celebrate with an ice cream that it is just one more 'chemo.' You just need a little patience, and it will be over in a few weeks. Soon you will see the light at the end of the tunnel."

June 21

The words were kind and encouraging, but I was full of gloom, unable to forget for a minute the effects of the CMF on my body: the nausea, the sinus congestion, the aches in all my bones, the restless nights, the abnormal imagery, the immense fatigue that lingered so long, and finally the weight gain due to limited activities, to changed metabolism, and to increased appetite. I had gained 13 pounds, an enormous amount for me, 10% exactly of my usual body weight. I could not wear several of my favorite clothes. I could not tolerate belts, panty hose, or underpants pressing, however slightly, on my stomach or my waist. The feeling of being changed bodily, altered in so many ways, gave me a persistent, unremitting feeling of not being myself, not being in tune with my own body. A certain mood of inhabiting a foreign land, of not being able to recognize all the messages sent about me by my body, alienated me in a manner I can barely describe.

These perceptions changed during the interval in each cycle between the moment of the injections and the beginning of the third week, after the last symptoms caused by the drugs (swollen eyelids, corneal irritation, and constant tearing) had disappeared. During that last week I was able to sense some reviving, though weak, signals of my old body. It was at this point of self-recognition that I felt the strongest hatred for the drugs that so altered me. I did not want to go once more and start the alienation all over again. It was repugnant to my whole being. I knew, however, I had to go. My life depended on it. Cancer is not an illness to play with. Invasive cancer knows no limits. Either the drugs kill the invasive cells capable of traveling enormous bodily distances to find a place to grow wildly, unchecked, or the cells kill you in their unrelenting reproductive march.

I wanted to live. The decision had been made in me and had been approved by me. I wanted to complete my life, to close the cycle of my path on earth in a more natural manner after I had finished some work I still had to do. I felt that some aspects of my personal life needed maturing, ripening of some fruits; that if left as they were now they would not render what they could have rendered. I was thinking about personal relations and work: some unfinished dialogues that might require a long time, particularly with my distant relatives. I did not want to die without reencountering them in whatever way possible. I was also thinking about work, some discoveries I was in the process of making, papers I was writing, and my teaching, which was now acquiring new depth and wider horizons. I wanted to die ripe, having done my job. I knew that my wishes might not be fulfilled. The metastases do not ask you how close you are to finishing your work when they make their decision to colonize your liver, your bones, your lungs, or your brains. They do as they please.

My only weapon—this *was* a war—was to kill any traveling metastatic cell before it reached its destination. To live meant to use so powerful a weapon that no enemy survived: a true holocaust of a cursed race of cells.

I understood as clearly as a besieged and starved city understands that without the surrender of the enemy there is nothing but death.

I had to go for my last injection against the clamor of all of me because I knew that I—the thinking woman—knew better than that poor naive *me* who did want to live and enjoy the pleasures of work and friendship with uninformed innocence. I knew that the wishes of *me* were not even thinkable without my suffering this treatment.

Three days before the injection I had a visit with my oncologist. Dr. Nagle welcomed me with his friendly and playful manner. I needed his easygoing style. He was a good ten years younger than I. That pleased me because I felt that he could remain my doctor-companion until my death. It was a selfish reason but good for both of us.

He asked me how I was. I said dryly, knowing his sense of humor, "Well enough, considering the *mis*treatment I am getting." He answered in kind, "Not good." We sat down. I had made it a habit to bring with me all the things I had to report and all my questions written down on a little notebook that the hospital's volunteers had given me as a gift.

He said, "What is in your list?" While I talked, he began to transcribe my health report into the record like a dutiful scribe. We talked matter-of-factly about symptoms, things to check, blood counts, fatigue, weight gain, side effects, changes in the future. The report of my symptoms was within predictable limits for people in my situation. He said I was doing as well as I could while receiving chemotherapy. I laughed at his giving me a good report card and said, "Summa cum laude in chemotherapy." We both laughed. He then examined me, carefully exploring the entire surface of my body to detect messages I might have missed in my self-report. He found nothing abnormal. I got dressed, and we talked about *me*.

That is what I liked most about him. He was *my* doctor. The doctor of *all of me*, not just a cancer fighter or a body keeper, but a man concerned with a woman who found herself ill with cancer. We talked about my feelings, my worries, my immediate future. The visit lasted 30 minutes and was very satisfactory. I left with the feeling of being in good hands, understood as a person, respected as a human being in physical and psychical distress.

The visit lifted my spirits to face the last injection on Friday. I finished my work in the early afternoon and loaded up my pocketbook with my two weapons against the metallic taste I so feared: the bottle of perfume and a few cookies.

All went as planned. Monique—who was nine months pregnant and had decided to work to the very end—hid the syringe from me, I let the cookies melt in my mouth while inhaling the perfume I had placed on a piece of gauze. I did not feel the metallic taste or the smell. Monique chatted with me quietly about this being the end of the chemotherapy and gently told me that I should be patient because it would take a while until I felt really well again. She said that two months was the average time. We also talked a bit about the plastic surgery that was to take place six weeks after this last treatment. So it was that before I had time to worry some more, the end had come. I had completed the course of treatment, and it had gone well. Monique and I said good-bye and promised to see each other in the oncology unit when I came from my regular check-up visit to the oncologist. We both smiled, thinking at the same time that it would be better if I did not need her any more. We did not say it. We just parted with good wishes for each other.

Now I had to face three more weeks of feeling ill and fatigued before I could begin to plan to return to more normal days. There were things to consider about my health that still needed care. I had been left without a single sex hormone in my body. The oncologist and I had agreed that vaginal changes would occur: dryness, atrophy, itching. There was also a need to attend to the possibility of osteoporosis. For these two concerns I needed a gynecologist. I had lost mine just a few months before I discovered the lump in my breast. Rather than return to Dr. Marcus, the gynecologist who had diagnosed my cancer, and who after all her promises never called again, it seemed better now to go to someone connected with the hospital where I was being treated. I therefore decided to ask the oncologist for the name of a woman gynecologist he knew and could recommend. This new consultation felt to me like the beginning of a restoration, of repair to a damaged old structure.

When I called for an appointment, I once more found a dictator for a secretary. She interrogated me about my referring doctor as though I were planning to rob the office. She claimed I could not see the doctor in less than two months, and then only after she checked with my referring doctor. Obviously she did not believe me. She said that she would call back. She never did. A few days later I called back and asked to speak directly with the gynecologist. The same secretary said that it was not possible. I asked her about her "checking on me." She informed me that she had talked to my oncologist and that what I had said about needing an appointment sooner than two months was true. Then, continuing with her dictatorial manner, she gave me, as a concession to her newly found truth, an appointment one month later. At that point, I committed the terrible error of asking her how old the gynecologist was because I wanted a woman not much younger than myself. That question set her afire. She went into a tirade about how inappropriate my question was and that she was not about to answer it. I had had it with her. I told her I was not about to play games with her and hung up.

I thought that she could have been a first-rate war criminal had she been born in Hitler's Germany. Her inclination to dominate, control, and humiliate seemed marvelously suited for a torturer but certainly was out of place for a medical secretary.

I was beginning now to learn that secretaries are like a Siegfried Line, an enormous line of resistance to prevent contact between doctor and patient. I wondered how they end up sitting at their secretarial desks. Certainly not all of them are bad. My surgeon's and plastic surgeon's secretaries were delightful and always helpful and willing to fetch a doctor for me. I calculate, however, that of the six doctors' secretaries I had to deal with during this period, two were helpful, the other four seemed always to be grouchy, dealt with me as though I were a nuisance, and seemed to be eager to postpone my contact with the doctor as long as they could. According to my private statistics, only a meager 33% are good medical secretaries. My experiences lead me to believe that there is a need to educate them better – they cannot possibly be as mean as they seem – to help them understand how critical their first contact with a patient is. They need to understand that they are part and parcel of the medical treatment itself and that there is a lot of therapeutic work to be found in the kind words of a medical secretary.

Dr. Myrna Katz, the gynecologist, was a woman slightly older than I, who did not remember who had referred me to her. I told her the story, and we got to our business. She was matter-of-fact about my troubles. We talked about strategies to protect vaginal tissues that needed extra care now that hormones, their natural nutrients, were not available to them. We talked about the ways in which I could be helped. She confirmed what I knew, that in the seven months since my last hormone pill some demonstrable damage had taken place. She recommended some practices of vaginal care that could compensate for the structural changes. For my probable osteoporosis she recommended exercise, particularly walking and a diet high in calcium.

She accepted that I had to decide whether or not I would keep her as my gynecologist. She said that she knew I had to decide whether or not I felt comfortable with her. I appreciated her position and told her that I would return for a second visit when necessary. She said that a yearly checkup was all I needed. Then she asked me to obtain the records from my previous gynecologist so that she could have a full knowledge of my gynecological history. I promised to bring them with me at the time of my next consultation.

I left her office with mixed feelings. It was sad and worrisome to have confirmed the deleterious effects of the lack of hormones in my body and in my genitals. It meant learning that I had entered a decline in my life that was irreversible. I would never again have a hormonally supported body. To protect my organs I had to use artificial methods and be faithful to them. I had to do what nature had always done but could no longer do. I felt the weight of the change that had occurred in me, and sadness came upon me. I also felt that Dr. Katz had given me clear directions and a way of dealing with the inevitable. Furthermore, she had explicitly indicated that she was willing to help, to ally herself with me in this limited battle of containment, and that I could call her anytime if I had any worries. I felt she was my ally and appreciated how good it was to have one at this time when I was feeling beaten down and on the path of unavoidable decline.

June 28

The three weeks after the treatment went well. I did not vomit or experience the metallic taste. All the other symptoms were there. The fatigue was more intense than usual and the nausea more persistent. The knowledge that I had no more treatments and that after three weeks I would continue to improve gave me a dim hope. I could not be cheerful because I was still dwelling in my body's trembling house.

All my friends, local friends and others from far, far away, called to celebrate the end of my trial. I felt like a performer of sorts, a marathon runner who had crossed the winning line and was staggering in front of a cheering crowd. They had accompanied me along the long road, faithfully giving me courage each time I needed it. All of them wanted to celebrate. I asked to postpone the celebration until I had a body that could dance again and stay up late at night. Then we could have many intimate and big celebrations in honor of my health and their faithful friendship.

By coincidence my friends Robin and Larry, who live 12 hours away from where I live, had to come to town for some ceremonies at their daughter's college. Robin, a handsome, dark-haired, slight woman, had witnessed her mother's death from cancer and had had breast cancer herself. Larry's mother had died a horrible death in a nursing home. They both had been acquainted with grief for a long time. Larry, a fellow physician, was beside himself when he learned I had breast cancer. We had been friends for many years and had shared precious moments of self-disclosure. Their affectionate response as soon as they heard came in tender words of courage to face the horrifying mastectomy. The first weekend after my discharge from the hospital Larry had come to visit me to "tell you everything you need to know about breast cancer."

He arrived on that day seven months ago at 10:00 A.M. and left at 4:00 P.M. We talked about every aspect of the illness's horror, from the fear of death and bodily destruction to all I had to do to live and live well. Larry could not contain his tears. So we cried together while we talked and also laughed, our faces covered with tears.

After lunch, as I was lying down on the living room couch, Larry was pacing back and forth crying. Suddenly he saw a man passing by. He shouted, "Do you see that man there walking happily?" It was a rhetorical question. Because I was lying down I could not see the man. "Well," he continued, "do you know what the difference is between him and you?" He dried his tears. "No, Larry," I said, "I don't." His voice reached a high pitch of rhetorical conviction, "He does not know he could die, and you do. Do you understand that? He could be dead tonight. Look at the passengers of the TWA plane crash. Where are they? They didn't think they could die. They went for a vacation. Where are they now? In the grave. Where are you now? Here," and he pointed at me with his right index finger, while drying his tears with his left hand.

I was moved by the sincerity and depth of his own pain for me. His words were imprinted on me like the voice of God himself. I have repeated them every day, while feeling all over again the emotion evoked by his impassioned deliverance of hopeful tidings.

Today, seven months later, we were remembering that intense moment and were laughing together at what we had shared so seriously then.

Robin had been very faithful to me, sending me a cheerful card each week with a small sentence of sober encouragement. She had also called on the telephone and shared with me what she had felt, what her dreams and her fears had been while she watched her mother's struggles with cancer and her own ordeal with breast cancer. It was a most generous act to appoint herself as a sweet companion in my prolonged tribulation.

Today we had a better mood. Their last child had just got settled in college, and they were beginning to experience the feelings of the empty nest syndrome. We talked about the children, their growing up, and the future life of a couple who have sent their fledglings into the world and who now have to make a new life together. We talked about eating habits, going out more, visiting children dispersed throughout the U.S.A. We rejoiced that they could now come to my town more frequently and stay with me. To celebrate all these milestones, we had dinner together at my house and crowned it with a delicious dessert of grapes, kiwis, and strawberries.

We realized that we were marking endings and beginnings. Robin said that now I was entering the third phase of the process: returning to a more normal life, to a healthier body, unencumbered by the urgency of the treatment or the illness itself. She predicted that I would perceive the implications and consequences of having had cancer for the rest of my life.

We talked about having a very clear hierarchy of values, appreciating the time at hand, acquiring a sober view about money, competition, and social success. We three felt that cancer, painful and frightening an illness as it was, had brought me to a major confrontation with myself and the meaning of my life. Robin had done her psychic work about the horrors of her mother's sufferings and had found peace, but not without pain, fear, and regrets.

I understood clearly. It was now my turn. In this third stage of my cancer episode, I had to face the entirety of my life's adventure with integrity and courage and let the fact of having cancer — or having *had* cancer, as one of my oncologist friends wanted me to phrase it — permeate my life, be integrated into it as part of who I am.

Robin and Larry left, and I went to bed exhausted and pleased, preoccupied, and overwhelmed. I felt that my new life's task – even though different from what it had been – was not less demanding than what I had already gone through. I knew, however, that if I was to preserve my psychic and moral integrity I had to do it.

The airwaves seemed to have picked up my thoughts because the following day I received a note from the social worker of the oncology department inviting me to join a support group for women with breast cancer.

I called her back, and we chatted amiably for a few minutes. She explained that the group was informal. Once a week people got together to talk about their experiences and about things that worried them and tiptoed around other experiences that they were afraid of talking about. We then talked about me, the friends who were helping me, my situation as a physician known in the community. After pondering all those factors, we agreed that it was better for me not to attend the group but to keep on obtaining all the help and support I already had. I felt respected by her and respected her judgment, and it gave me peace that I had not blindly rejected an open hand extended to me.

5

Reshaping

July 5

My next move was to have my last presurgery visit with the plastic surgeon to decide about the details of what was to be done. I looked forward to the visit because it meant the beginning of the end of this lengthy episode of illness and mourning.

On the surface, the visit was routine: a final checkup and the last discussion about all the details. In the depths of myself the sea waves of intense personal and bodily feelings were reaching high levels and were falling full force on the shore of my awareness.

I had formed a habit of looking directly into the mirror that reflected my naked body. On my left side, I had a high and delicate hill of white flesh surrounding its darker milk fountain. The skin was shiny, the vessels underneath, transparent, the shape firm and proud.

On my right side, there was a scar crossing the space of the absent breast. Reddish, almost purple, its diagonal went from near the sternum to the armpit. There the linear scar became a deep, hollow pit the bottom of which rested on my ribs. I could fit four of my fingers up to their second phalanxes into it. Under the skin I had the plastic expander full of saline solution. It felt foreign and external to me. It gave me a feeling of constraint and oppression, comparable to what I thought Roman soldiers must have felt under the heavy coating of their bronze pectoral plates. The skin of the breast area, armpit, arm, and a small section of the forearm had a diminished, dull sensitivity because they had lost the connecting nerves capable of giving them the subtle language of the flesh. From now on, that sector of myself would be like a retarded child, appreciative of tender caresses but incapable of discerning the nuances of a true dialogue. I knew that this change was forever, as long as I lived.

The shame of having a damaged body is unavoidable. Mine had been a proud, efficient, elastic, well-disposed body, a body I loved and enjoyed and liked to parade around discreetly but proudly. Now I was ashamed that people would notice the fake breast, the acrylic breast under my clothes, that they would notice the different shapes of my flesh breast and my fake breast. I worried about clothes and tried to select them for their capacity to hide an anatomy that was the source of shame and humiliation. That was not the end of my bodily concerns. The 13 pounds I had gained was a very large amount for a person who had kept the same weight for 25 years. I could not wear most of my clothes. I did not want to buy new clothes, for I knew that when I became well again I was going to lose the foreign pounds.

The absence of hormones and the disregulation of my autonomic system due to the chemotherapy kept my body on an unpredictable see-saw of feeling very hot (hot flashes with profuse perspiration) and very cold, to the point that I could not warm up without the use of an electric heating pad, even when the temperature outside was 84°.

I had no energy. I had always been a brisk walker, dashing from one place to another with great pleasure. Now I walked like a turtle—heavily, slowly, stopping to catch my breath. Stairs, which I used to love (they are good for your figure and heart), were now like a local train itinerary. I had to stop at several points, huffing and puffing like an old-fashioned locomotive.

Then there were the darker secrets of my ashamed body: the skin changes, bone changes, genital tissue changes due to the absolute absence of any sex hormone.

Finally, there were the other bodily miseries of everyday life that had preceded the cancer: a progressive osteoarthritis with a poorly functioning shoulder and a thyroid gland that could not carry its burden and had to be supplemented with thyroid pills.

This collection of bodily misfunctions required constant attention. I realized one day that I was the only one in charge of the assorted parts of myself. The surgeon now cared for the final healing of the wound. The plastic surgeon had eyes only for my breast. My oncologist covered the spectrum by surveying my general health. My gynecologist checked the bottom half of my anatomy – the breast having been surrendered to the oncologist and radiologist (mammograms) for gynecological atrophy and other miseries. All the doctors were kind and helpful, but it was only my persistent questioning that brought about some options and potential solutions for me as a living woman.

I had been reflecting about these matters for a while when I discovered a tremendous longing within me. I wanted my pediatricians back , the two of them, the man of my childhood and the woman of my early teens. I wanted them to care for me *now* as they had for me and my siblings by assuming full responsibility for our welfare from head to toe, always anticipating what the child needed first and then returning to the child her healthy body.

Dr. Martin Pellerin, my first pediatrician, was a very tall, thin-legged man with broad, stooping shoulders, a deep voice emerging from well-formed lips, which were shaped for commanding and full words. He had a big head with premature white hair flowing around deep blue eyes. In an age when doors were not locked, he would knock, open the door, and say very loudly, "Who is sick in this house?" Even if I was very sick, I always had enough voice to answer him with great intensity. "It is me, Dr. Pellerin, Madeleine." He would then greet my parents, come to my room, throw a piercing look at me from head to toe – I believed he could see everything – and then ask my mother for something to warm up his hands, his stethoscope, and anything else that was to be in contact with my body. While warming up, he would repeat his maxim: "A doctor must not touch a child with cold hands or instruments."

When he had warmed up, tools and all, he would come to my bed and, holding me by the shoulders, help me stand on the bed so that our heads were at the same level. If I was too weak, he held me. If not, he would put his big and gentle hands on the sides of my face, look into my eyes, smile, and say, "How are you, little lady?" I could feel that he meant the question as more than a social amenity. He would then explore my expression, caress my hair, and pinch my cheeks, his face adapting to the message. If I was very sad, he had a kind silent smile; if I was in better spirits, he complimented me about something, my nose, my curls, my school work. This done, the scene was set for two very unequal friends to cooperate in the examination. I trusted him totally. I knew that he loved me and that he was a thorough diagnostician and a very well-informed clinician. The examination was always very serious because he totally concentrated in his work.

Then he would reflect silently for a while, reach some conclusions, and finally write not only the prescription but all the details of the physical care I needed. He read those to my mother, clarifying every detail about what to do and how to do it. The task completed, he would return to the original ceremony of standing me up and looking me straight in the eye. He would then tell me how I was going to feel, about the bitter things I had to swallow, and when he was coming back. At that point, holding my face in his hands once more, he would say, "Bye, little lady." As soon as he left, I was three quarters cured. His attentions to me, his conveying that he was in charge and was going to do a good job in helping me, gave me a fantastic devotion to whatever he said I had to do. Bitter pills could be taken almost without effort because I took them not for myself but for him.

He provided a marvelous resting place between people where you could truly lean on the shoulders of a good Samaritan who knew how to carry you to your healing point. I loved him with a mixture of joy (of which he had plenty), respect, and tenderness. There was something very tender about him, even though it was well known that he could turn into a ferocious tiger if he saw a child who was not being properly taken care of. He could boss the parents around with his powerful voice and say appalling things to colleagues who had missed a diagnosis. I also loved him because I knew that while he was there in charge of me I did not have to worry. *He* was truly in charge and would not miss a detail, however small, that was needed to make me comfortable. I am sure that I became a doctor to be to others what he had been to me and my siblings.

July 12

I also used as a model a woman doctor who saved the life of my little brother after several pediatricians had said there was nothing else to do for him. She was different from Dr. Pellerin. Dr. Martha Calder was a soft-spoken, dark-haired, middle-sized woman in her early thirties. She was timid and unassuming. She worked with slow grace and spoke softly with well-pondered words. She had deep, large, brown eyes, full of melancholy. She would examine you first with her melancholic eyes, surveying all of you from the tip of your soul to the tip of your toes. Then she would sit down next to your bed and let you tell her about your aches and pains. She listened, seriously asking a question here, another there, or she would point with her fingers at the source of pain. When she seemed to understand the nature of your complaints and your fears, she would get up, bend over you, and check you all over with the fingers of a pianist eliciting notes from the keyboard. During her careful examination I used to feel I was a very precious and special being, a certain living piece of art that had to be restored delicately to its original shape and beauty.

When the whole examination was over, she would think for a few minutes and then, opening her melancholic face into a big smile, would announce her diagnosis in simple, colloquial terms. She always crowned her brief speech with a dramatically comical remark , "You have no guts; they are all inflamed. We'll take care of it all. I won't let a lousy inflammation knock you down. Get gutsy and take the bitter things I'll give you. You'll be better soon."

I used to imagine a sort of pact between Dr. Calder and myself to combat that impertinent invader called gut's inflammation or paratyphoid infection. I am sure that my immune system could hear the words of that "we'll take care of it" as a command to summon every soldier lymphocyte to fierce combat. I had already begun to feel better as soon as she left the room smiling.

What I liked most about Drs. Pellerin and Calder was their joyful, quiet enthusiasm to join me in my wish to get well, while it was obvious that it was they who were in firm command of a situation I could not control. I was a child. They were big doctors who did not make me feel small and obnoxious because I complained. Instead they called me – the healthy part of me – to join them as a trusted assistant to help out in the healing process. I was always so pleased with their trust in me that I myself made a conscious effort to get better *for* them, to show them that *I* deserved the trust they had placed on *me*.

My longings for the bygone pediatricians increased with my growing awareness that in our modern system of medicine no one is in charge of the person as patient. While I was in the midst of these reflections, reality proved them correct. The events themselves were prosaic and banal in the way that true evil can be banal.

It all started with my last visit before surgery to Dr. Keily who was to give me a final checkup and discuss with me the details of the surgical procedures and the expected results.

July 19

The visit was as friendly as it had always been. Dr. Keily had been operating all day long, and he seemed very tired. His secretary had canceled all other patients but was unable to reach me. He came late and apologized for the delay. We talked in a quiet and careful manner about the details of the surgery. I was concerned about the deep pit I had near the axilla. It brought the skin in contact with the ribs, leaving a deep fold. We discussed the possibility of filling it up with some fat tissue. He did not guarantee good results but promised to do the best he could. He was thinking so deeply, with his eyes half closed, imagining what to do and how to do it, that I could almost see what he was imagining doing.

We then talked about breast size. I had always been a 34B, but after surgical menopause ten years earlier, when I was given the routine dosage of estrogen and progesterone, the hormones promoted my breasts to a size 36C, almost D. Dr. Keily was now looking intently at my left, healthy breast. I could see him mulling the best course of action for the last time. He said it was not advisable to use a large implant, that it was better for my future to have my normal breast reduced to size 34 or smaller to match the implant. The reason was that a weighty breast would tend to drop more easily than a lighter one. In the course of time the implant would remain in place, and the level of my breasts on my chest would become uneven.

We discussed every pro and con in clear, simple sentences until we came to the joint decision that reducing the size of the normal breast and lifting it a little to match the height of the implant was the best course. My sense of humor intervened, and I heard my thought, "You'll be an adolescent after this breast lifting." I kept it to myself because Dr. Keily was still thinking and operating in his mind. When he finished the imaginary surgery, he turned to me and asked if there were other things to talk about. I mentioned that he had suggested the possibility of making a nipple of sorts. He said he had. I said he had mentioned two possibilities: to do it at the time of placing the implant or to do it later. I asked what were the pros and cons and what was his advice on the matter. He again entered the world of imaginary surgery and , emerging out of it in a few minutes, said that he could do it with "the little piece of nipple skin" – the alreola of my normal breast – "that we usually throw away." An indignant roar raised within me when I heard him talk about "throwing away" such a precious part of my skin. I felt insulted and indignant. I realized, however, that he had no intention of offending me. He was only carrying out his mental surgery. I calmed myself down without revealing my inner storm. He continued, "With that bit I can make you a new nipple." I forgave him at this point because he was not throwing the precious bit away. Instead he was going to make use of it on the other side. He went on, "Now," and he looked at me, "you must know that it is not possible to place the two nipples at a perfectly even height. There could be 1 centimeter difference between them." I said that I did understand the technical difficulties and that it would not be a problem for me because I knew it would not be noticeable unless someone went around with a tape, measuring me for symmetry.

All was now in order, or so it seemed. He came out of his operating dream, smiled broadly, asked me to finalize details with his secretary, Cora, and, shaking hands while smiling, said in his usual lighthearted manner, as though we were going to a resort together, "I'll see you then."

Cora and I had become friendly with each other out of the simple habit of biweekly visits. She was very pretty, eager to help and efficient. She, too, had a light touch in her voice and manner. She was waiting for me when I came out of the office. I told her that two months earlier Dr. Keily and I had set up my surgery for August 10. I asked her to check that everything was in order. Cora looked at me, paused for a minute and said, "I don't have you scheduled for surgery. That day is completely booked, and we don't have any openings in the operating room for a month." She plunged into the book and came out of it saying, "The best I can do is to see if some patients can change their elective surgery and make room for you. But it would be one or two weeks later."

I was so shocked that I could barely talk. I said, almost to myself, in total disbelief, "We talked about Thursday, the 10th of August, two months ago, and we repeated the date each time I met with him. He said it was all right."

She looked at me. "He does not operate on Thursdays." My bewilderment reached the point of muteness, a most unusual condition for me.

Finally I said, "Listen. I have arranged my entire life around the time we agreed upon. I gave Dr. Keily a complete schedule of my plans each time I came, so that he would know how I was organizing my surgery and my postsurgical care. I can't believe what you are telling me. I just can't."

She became defensive for the first time. She said, "You didn't tell me."

I got furious. "He forgot to tell you. It is *his* fault, Dr. Keily's fault. I tell you when *he* tells *me* to talk to you. I am not your boss."

She retreated and said in a more friendly way, "I'll see what I can do. I can't give you the date you have, August 10. I can only give you a week later."

I told her what trouble that would create for me. I had carefully orchestrated the care of my patients, the household help, the friends coming from abroad, tickets, reservations, life plans; all of these would have to be changed by *me*. Finally I collapsed and blurted, "This is total disaster. I don't know what to do."

It was very late now, long past her time to leave for the day. She said, "I'll do the best I can." I thanked her and apologized for keeping her so late. She said, "It is all right," and left in a hurry.

I was furious to the extreme and completely bewildered. I truly did not know what to do, an unusual predicament for me. In my anger, humiliation, the feeling of being a piece of surgical meat, a number on an operating list, it dawned on me that Dr. Keily had never *listened* to all of my careful planning. His dreaming surgery—his five-year-old playing with mud pies—had not made room for the impact of his actions on me, his plaything. I was so angry, so frustrated that I felt I was not fit to drive, having to control physical fatigue and fury at the same time. I sat in my car, talking to myself and hitting the wheel while chewing my words, "Bastard, selfish bastard." The raging words, spit out of my mouth like vitriolic acid, calmed me down enough to drive home.

I had just sat down in despair when the phone rang. It was my friend Doris, a surgeon herself, who was calling to check if all was right with me. I began telling her about a mishap on the schedule. She blurted out, "Your surgery is on August 10. I have known that myself for two months." "No, no, Doris," I said, "It is not going to be." She became indignant and ordered me to call the surgeon at his home right away and tell him to fix it regardless of what he had to do. She knew, being a surgeon herself, that one can always find space in the operating room. Her indignation helped me to calm down. I obeyed her orders, aware that if I had not been so furious, feeling so let down, so totally ignored, I would have thought of it myself.

I called, and he answered the phone in his playful voice. I told him that there was no room for me in his schedule after we had planned every detail for two months, that I didn't know where to start if I had to change the date. He said with the same light voice, as though he had discovered some minor fault in himself, "I forgot. I didn't tell Cora." I didn't know what else to say. He seemed totally unaware of my distress. I repeated, "I don't know where to start if I have to change my plans." He said, without apologizing or compunction, "Don't change anything. I'll talk to Cora on Monday." I reminded him that I was pressed for time because I could not in only a few days make all the changes I had to make. The surgery was now four weeks away. He repeated, "I'll talk to Cora. She'll call you."

Monday came and Cora did not call. I called her at the end of the day. Dr. Keily had again forgotten to talk with her about the surgical schedule. She, however, had been frantically calling other patients to make room for me. I asked her to talk with him at once. She said she would call on Tuesday. She did not. I called her. She said she was waiting for some patients to call back to give me a date a week later. I insisted that I had to know very soon to reorchestrate my entire life. I repeated that my entire life would be in chaos if I had to change the date. She said she would do what she could.

On Wednesday she did not call. I had to inform one of my patients of possible changes in my schedule. She was a very sick woman and unexpected changes on my part would bring her to the edge of psychosis. On Thursday Cora still had not called. I called her, whereupon she informed me in a casual way that Dr. Keily was trying to swap operating room time with another plastic surgeon to have my operation at the time originally scheduled. I thanked her and then said I had to get something off my chest. I told her that the greatest error of my life was to trust Dr. Keily and not to double check everything myself. She said nothing.

I meant what I said. Something final and irrevocable had happened between Dr. Keily, Cora, and me. I could no longer feel that I was a person, least of all that I was a woman overburdened by illness, exhaustion, fear of cancer, and the absence of a family to help me out. I felt that I could no longer afford to be a trusting patient. I was dealing with technicians and bureaucrats, technically perfect in performing bits of surgery on sleeping bodies. Even Cora, friendly as she appeared to be, did not show an ounce of concern about the havoc Dr. Keily had created for me. She talked like the mail clerk that has to fit letters and pieces of mail into slots. When she found no slot for me, I was handled with bureaucratic nonchalance until by some coincidence of factors I could be pushed into a space of sorts.

The worst feeling was the sense of utter impotence. I imagined dropping dead in front of them and her calling up the morgue to pick my body up while she kept transcribing his notes. I counted as a mastoplasty case—one of many, but one who was particularly troublesome because I could not be moved like a chess piece without protesting very loudly.

I could not change surgeons. Nobody would take me. He was one of the most reputable in town. I did trust his skill, so I made my decision with tears and with rage. Then, when he fixed my body and had me finished as a technical success ("mastectomy 2,173, female 54, Caucasian, successful operation"), I would be printed as a number in one of his papers. The paper would not mention my anguish or his disregard of me.

Just before the surgery, my mood changed to one of resigned sadness for a medical world that no longer has patients but only diseases, procedures, techniques and diagnostic codes. Men and women, children and old people fall through the holes of the medical net like small fish from the fisherman's net.

The time came for the preadmission interview. The head of nursing mailed me a questionnaire asking about all sorts of things, from my sleeping habits to my religious beliefs. Each question indicated that it was asked so that they could tailor their services to my needs. I answered, after my experience with Dr. Keily, with the devotion of a child writing to Santa Claus. The paranoid in me laughed. "You," it said, "you with your silly hopes. You are going to a teaching hospital, and they are doing research about patients' habits and needs." *Me* said softly, "Maybe not. Maybe they mean it." And I, the woman physician in charge of myself, thought that to be equidistant between hope for the best and paranoid watchfulness for the worst was the only place to be.

August 2

I was still in the midst of my storm when I received a letter from my friend Patricia, a professor of international relations at a midwestern university. The letter informed me that she had just had surgery for cancer of the colon. They had resectioned a portion of the large intestine, and the surgeon had found that the cancer had not penetrated the intestinal wall. There was no metastasis in the lymph nodes. Her doctors assured her that she was totally cured. She had lost a lot of weight and was having difficulty eating. She was doing the best she could to recover, to come back to everyday life, after the terrible fright of having cancer and the bodily devastation of the surgery. She was coming to my area, where she had lived before, to continue her convalescence and wanted to be sure she could see me because she felt she could talk with me about her feelings of fear and of suffering. She ended the letter with a sentence most unusual for her, "I curse this cancer and spit in its face." It sounded like the bravery of someone very frightened. Besides, I could not help noticing that her cancer was a person with a face. I instantly asked myself what my own cancer was like. I realized that my cancer was not a person, not something with malice and ill will. It was nature derailing, blindly multiplying, with the destructive innocence of bacteria or viruses: the frantic growth, the vital spur of misguided cells that my body did not know how to stop.

I could only see in my cancer a fact of life, a component of the risk of being alive. I could not unravel its ultimate meaning. I did not feel it made any sense to ask, "Why me?" because the question assumes that I should not be subjected to the ordinary vicissitudes of life and death. The question for me was always, "What now?" I could not personalize my cancer, deal with it as though it were a person. I was therefore bewildered by Patricia's hating and defiant remark. I realized that she needed to say it for reasons that escaped me. She had her way, I had mine, to face a death sentence. Her doctors had told her that her sentence had been commuted. My doctors had said to me that they could not say anything. The statistics gave me a 75% chance to be alive five years from now. That was all.

Patricia had included her phone number in the letter as an unstated request for a call. I had to decide whether or not to tell her about my own cancer. It was a very painful decision to make. It involved my honesty, my respect for her reality, my fear that she would find it impossible to keep my cancer confidential when she had told everybody – so she said in her letter – about her own. I had to consider her point of view too. She seemed taken over by her condition. We were friends, but not that close. What would she and I gain by my saying, "I too have cancer." Finally, I talked to a couple of common friends who knew her very well. They all were worried about her and her way of handling her condition. She seemed to them terrified of what had happened to her and unable to acknowledge that she was frightened. My friends' advice was that I should not tell her about myself. I felt guilty and disloyal, like a real liar, but I decided to call her and talk only about her, as though everything was well with me. The conversation centered on all the details of her surgery and recovery. She did not ask about me or my health, and I was grateful that I did not have to use convoluted words to avoid a direct lie.

Finally, a few days later she came to town, and we went together for a short walk around the neighborhood. She walked slowly to keep pace, and, I, unbeknownst to her, walked slowly to make sure I did not get short of breath.

We started the conversation gently. She spoke of her caring friends – she has no family – and all the people who had rallied to her side to help her out. She was walking a bit bent over as though she still feared the surgical wound would open up. We laughed a little about that. Then, much to my anguish, she told her whole story, indicating that only those who have been there can know what it is like: the need to check everything, to see what doctor does what, get their opinions about options, diagnosis, prognosis, etc., etc. I was feeling as rotten as I could feel about my not telling her about my cancer, but I kept sensing that my decision was right.

Then, suddenly, her words jolted me. I knew that what the doctors had said was correct. Hers had been a localized lesion, and she was free of cancer. But she was now saying that she had to go for another sigmoidoscopy for the doctors to see *if there were new growths.* I looked at her and asked her to repeat what she meant. She did mean what I had heard. I explained to her that the procedure was a routine follow-up unrelated to new growths. I could not get my point across. She believed herself still sick with cancer and expected it to continue its destructive march on her. I felt fearful for her. Then, resorting to my medical authority, I repeated that the doctors might want to check that the surgical procedure was functioning normally, rather than check for new cancer. She said that she was relieved after hearing my explanation, and, to a point, I could see she was. I could sense, though, that she did not believe she was free of cancer and was terrified of it.

For my own peace of mind I asked her to tell me whatever was written on the record. She had a photocopy of it at home and had memorized it. From what she said, I could do nothing but conclude that the whole cancer had been removed and that she was in fact free of cancer and with a negligible possibility of a reappearance. Her cancer was the type that does not metastasize. I said all this to her. She listened and then responded by saying that she had started a most rigorous diet to protect herself against cancer and that she believed in the evidence that cancer could be contained by dieting. I told her she had nothing to contain. She insisted that she could get another cancer, that we all have to diet to destroy cancerous cells in our body.

My anguish doubled. I not only felt like a deceiver and a liar but also like an outsider, someone who, having been there and still being there, nevertheless could not enter her experience. She now had cancer in her soul, and this new cancer had begun to dominate her life and was poisoning her soul and our friendship. I realized to my sorrow that I had failed to reach her. The wish to tell her about myself was very intense. Now, not telling her was not an option but an obligation. She had entered the long, dark tunnel of fear, and I could not help her. I had neither an invitation nor access to the obscure regions of her mind where cancer was a personal offender who had to be cursed and spat on.

I felt terribly lonely and sad because secretly I wanted to say, "We had cancer," and to feel we were together in a shared tragedy, an ordinary human tragedy, now extraordinary because it was ours. I could not enter her world of self-absorption even if I wanted company in my pain.

Patricia's other friends called me later. They worried as much as I did about her dark fear of a hidden enemy.

We talked more about her and about me. I was still afraid, but not of a dark destruction. I was afraid and sad about the prospects of an incomplete life. I was frightened of prolonged illness and pain without a family, in an impersonal nursing home. I had seen the infamous nursing homes for the poor in Washington. The sister of a friend of mine had died a horrible death, burned by scalding water in the bathtub in a nursing home. I had visited senior professors in nursing homes and heard them being called "Mike, dear." The memories awoke my worst fears: the loss of dignity, the loss of myself in the unmade bed of a hospital or a nursing home where people would call me by my first name only and would be more concerned about my bowel movements than about the fact that I was living the last chapter of my life and wanted to exit as I had lived. Death is inevitable and necessary. It is a gift to be able to live one's own death. I had seen that in my medical practice in my early years. Living with dignity until one dies requires endless acts of self-protection in a society that is concerned only with its neat division of labors and organs and cannot afford to deal with complete human beings.

August 12

Now the time was drawing near for my so-called reconstruction surgery. It would be the last step of my first, and perhaps (that was the voice of hope) only, cancer episode, which I had begun eight months earlier with apparently healthy breasts. I had found a little lump on the right breast. I had a biopsy for it. It was diagnosed as "infiltrating carcinoma." I consulted frantically to decide what to do. We all agreed on what to do. I had a modified radical mastectomy. A week later the pathologist said I had two metastases. Everybody agreed that I had to have chemotherapy. I had eight courses of CMF every three weeks. I was supposed to lose my hair. I didn't. I gave up the wig. The plastic surgeon had placed in me a so-called expander, a plastic breastlike water bag that he injected once a week with 30 or 50 cc of saline solution. He filled it to 550 cc. It looked like a little mountain cut across by a surgical scar, ending in a deep pit under my arm. Now he had to take out the expander, put in the so-called implant (an amazing looking, breastlike plastic mass), make a nipple with a piece of the other nipple on my left side, reduce the size of my left breast, try to fill in the pit at the axilla, and then, after all that ordeal, I would be once more a double-breasted woman.

I laughed at the new woman to come, saying, "You'll be like a bionic woman: half human and half synthetic." One of my best friends, who knew my sense of humor, sent me a card with a blooming rose tree and two cut out paper roses inside saying "for your new blooming."

My mood was contradictory, oscillating. At moments I felt hopeful, feeling that all would be over and I could go on freely, at least for a few years, about the business of life. Another part of me, scared and superstitious could not believe that better days were about to come. I had—perhaps like Patricia—an obscure and unnamed fear of bad things about to happen. I was like a child holding tightly to the monster in the closet as a protection against other, unnamable fears.

I wanted it to be over, finally over, and yet I was afraid of its being over. As the day was drawing near, I was feeling the cloudy fear of having to live without thinking all the time about my physical condition. If I were to create a neologism I should say I was having a fear of not being preoccupied about my flesh, a "sarcophobia" or something like that.

I knew the surgery was simple, not really painful, and that nobody expected any complications. Now my mood moved in the other direction. I was in a hurry. I wanted it to be over. I wanted to be free, no longer fatigued, able to do what I wanted. I began to travel in my head. I took several exotic trips: to central China, to the Himalayas, to the jungles of Brazil. I also went to the highlights of Western civilization: Budapest, Paris, Rome. In between, I criss-crossed the lakes, mountains, and plains of Latin America. When I returned from my wild, imaginary trips I realized that I would have to wait a while to fully regain my stamina before I took even a far more modest trip. In fact, some close friends had invited me to convalesce in their house in another state, a four-hour trip. This simple reality brought my dreams to an end. The adventurous *me* gave way to the *me* in need of care and affection after the surgery. I felt disposed to entrust myself to my friends and their wish to pamper me and make me laugh.

August 9

Five days before the surgery I developed a mild sore throat and a head cold. A cold was a no-no. A printed order and directions form given to all preadmission patients said clearly and firmly, "If you develop a cold (cough, fever) or any other illness before your scheduled surgery, call your physician immediately at 831-9471. If you cannot contact your physician, call the Day Surgery Unit at 895-7325, Monday to Friday between 6:30 A.M. and 3:30 P.M."

The day before I had called the Day Surgery to check that all my preadmission tests, electrocardiogram, chest X-ray, and blood chemistry were normal and that the surgery would proceed as scheduled. I was assured that all was just fine and I was told to call the day before to check the time of morning to come to the hospital the day of the surgery.

My head cold had become an obsession and a nightmare. I worried it would not be over and that I would not be honest if I did not report it. In turn I worried about the last communication with my doctor. I feared that the surgery would be canceled, and I wanted so badly for it to be over. I feared that it would be carried out and that I would be very sick and everybody would blame me for not reporting the cold. I was afraid of the slightest draft of air or drop of rain. I watched every nuance of sensation in my head, every sneeze, every nose-blowing episode, a true cold-mania out of wish, fear, guilt, and a feeling of being alone with my dilemma. I had lost confidence in my doctor as a person, even though I fully trusted him as a surgeon. In view of the episode of his forgetting to schedule me, I did not feel I could count on him for a reasonable dialogue about a probable change of date for my surgery if I had to postpone. Finally, to come out of my obvious craziness and its effects on my poor friends, I decided to wait until 48 hours before the surgery. When the deadline arrived, a brilliant thought came to me. I called my friend Doris, the surgeon, and asked her to share the responsibility with me. In her most surgical manner, she cleared the air for me. She said, "1) If you do not have a fever, 2) if you do not have a cough, and 3) if you do not have too many secretions in your respiratory tract, there is no problem for the anesthesiologist. You can go without hesitation." My manic voices descended many decibels in my head but remained a little in the background, to return as a shout of guilt when my mild temperature after the surgery was attributed to some respiratory cause, "the most frequent cause of mild fever," as they said.

The day of the surgery there was bright sunlight, deep blue skies, and a delicious late spring air. My friend Gregory came faithfully at 7:00 A.M. to take me to the hospital. The surgery was scheduled for 9:00 A.M. The order of things required that I first go through paper work, bracelets, insurance papers, and other things. Finally, the nurse asked me to lie down on a stretcher and called the doctors. A friendly young resident started my I.V., not without saying that he was a bit intimidated because I was a doctor. Then the nurse, Marie, gave me every explanation I could need and told me she was going to be there when I woke up. Soon a bearded, middle-aged man with the looks of a Shakespearean English king came to greet me. He introduced himself as Dr. Hartvig ("King of Denmark," I said to myself).

He was obviously a kind and poised man. He proceeded immediately to supervise and teach the resident. I was not surprised to observe his manner and natural feeling of superiority. I felt pleased to be in the hands of a king-anesthetist. It was clear that he was not a regular member of Dr. Keily's team. He asked casually if Dr. Keily had seen me. I said he had not. I felt there was a certain tension there and could not help believing that Dr. Keily was angry because he had had to change his plans on account of me. My suspicion seemed confirmed when Dr. Hartvig said, "Dr. Keily told me that you are a psychiatrist." In my paranoia I heard, "Because you are a loony he has to operate today."

Dr. Keily appeared at that point but at a distance. I waved to him, trying to keep a certain friendship alive. He did not respond. This was very different from his warm handshaking and easy chatting of the time of the mastectomy, when he had been so gracious and easy going. This time he did not greet me at all, not even when I was wheeled into the operating room and he asked me to sit on the operating table so he could draw on my chest the outline of what he had to do. He drew with pencils of different colors as though he were painting a mural, and I was not there. He referred to me as "she" as he asked Dr. Hartvig if he had given me any premedication because he did not want "her to fall on me" while he was drawing on my chest. His words and manner reinforced my feelings of being treated like a thing, but I could still see his love of what he was doing and the fun he was having drawing his surgical plan on me in technicolor. His surgery was on, and I was definitely off, a nuisance he had to deal with to have his "mud pie fun."

I had become pretty philosophical after deciding that he could listen only to himself. As long as the operation was technically perfect, I was not going to ask for anything else from him. So I turned to Dr. Hartvig and the resident and fulfilled my need for human contact by exchanging a few simple words with them. The last one went to Dr. Hartvig, "I can feel you have given me something. I am falling asleep."

I woke up four hours later after two and a half hours of surgery and an hour and a half in the recovery room. I was greatly relieved that the last major hurdle was over and that now I had started the road to a more normal life. It did not matter that I feel some pain. Pain sooner or later subsides. The body, this amazing house in which we live, seems to have an endless capacity to restore itself. I knew I had to wait patiently for the pain to be over, rest as much as I could, and let my body do its healing work.

August 13

The normal pains were soon joined by something I did not expect because I had never had it after anesthesia: vomiting. It surprised me. Suddenly a wave of salivation (almost identical to the salivation that preceded the nausea after the chemotherapy) filled my mouth. Before I had time even to ponder what it was, my stomach sent up to my mouth a large amount of greenish, very acid fluid. It came out of me without my consent or participation. Fortunately, the nurses had placed a large plastic basin just at my hand's reach, and I did manage to catch in it the unexpected product of my stomach's eruption. The episode repeated itself several times for a good five hours. The nurses decided to keep my I.V. going and said that I could not drink or eat anything. Those restrictions and my burping episodes did not stop them from getting me out of bed and having me hold the I.V., like a prophet holding his staff, as I walked around the ward to exercise my anatomy. I was not inclined to like such an imposition, but after a little walking I could see that it helped me feel a bit better. It also improved my disposition, which at that point was becoming gloomy and irritable because I could see that I still had some side effects from the chemotherapy.

The promenade over, I lingered in bed as quietly as I could so as not to feel pain from my movements. The nurses were solicitous and eager for me to sleep without pain. They offered me pain medication and made every effort to make me comfortable. The person in charge during the evening shift was a young male nurse whose manner and deep melodic voice made me feel better at once. A wave of gratitude rose within me. I was extremely grateful that the entire staff of the unit and this young man in particular were all working—earning their living—by serving others with concern and good cheer.

Feeling cared for once more brought back the gratitude that, in spite of my distress with Dr. Keily, had overtaken me on entering the operating room, with its perfect order and immaculate cleanliness, and finding in it, in proper formation, like an army ready for combat, the whole surgical team. They were all dressed in green pants and surgical gowns and wore blue caps on their heads and white masks on their mouths. Only their eyes—like those of Arabian women—were visible. When I was being wheeled in they looked at me with a little spark of a different color in each person's eyes. They mumbled a short greeting and eased me onto the operating table, warning me that it was narrow and not to fall off the other side.

I looked at them. They were eight people altogether in surgical formation around me. Each had gone through many years of training, exams, work, internships, to have the right to be there in the surgical team. Each had learned to subordinate his or her actions to the team work under the joint leadership of the surgeon and the anesthetist. I felt that I was an extremely lucky person now to be the object of their care and technical skills. As a quick hypothetical exercise, I counted at least 80 years of experience at my service: surgeon, 20 years; anesthetist, 20 years; surgical resident, 5 years; anesthesia resident, 5 years; operating room nurse, 10 years; scrub nurse, 10 years; assistants, 5 years each. The moment I lay down, after Dr. Keily had finished his mural and just before going to sleep and saying my final words to Dr. Hartvig, all these thoughts gathered their impressive reality within me into a prayer of gratitude. Once more, following the steps of St. Francis, I thanked God for my brothers and sisters in the healing professions whose dedicated and faithful work was today, on this Thursday morning, at the service of helping me, and this afternoon and tomorrow and the day after tomorrow and each day until they retired from helping others like me. They would repeat their kind and welcoming gestures, which we patients need so much. I know I thought about them, the other seven in the team, to help myself to forgive Dr. Keily and to tolerate his rude behavior.

I am sure that these feelings of trust and gratitude helped me to have a most peaceful anesthesia for two and a half hours. Perhaps beyond oxygen and nitrous oxide, penthotal, brevitol, and other anesthetic substances, the presence of those people was like a mother's for her baby's sleep. I, like a grownup baby, entrusted myself to the good hands of the surgical team.

The morning after surgery I received the visit of the chief resident and his court. They were all cheerful and dashed in and out of my room, indicating with word and action that I "was doing well."

An hour later Dr. Keily came. He announced that all was fine and that I could go home right away. He seemed pleased with himself and his work on me. I was glad to see his satisfaction but not so pleased with his pushing me out of the hospital. "I am not ready to go," I said. "I live alone, and I am not ready to take care of myself."

The head nurse, who had followed him, came to my rescue. "Dr. Meldin did vomit a lot all night long. She has not eaten anything."

"I see," reflected Dr. Keily. "Well," he said to me, "you can go whenever you are ready, tomorrow, the day after tomorrow, any time you like." The light, playful voice had returned to him, and I felt pleased that he seemed to feel comfortable with me again.

He wanted to examine the surgical wound. I tried to see as much as I could. I saw something I had not expected. Encircling my nipples, the normal one and the new one for my implanted breast, I saw deep blue foam rubber that was stitched to my skin all around the nipples. I immediately thought, "I look like a cabaret dancer with flowers decorating her exposed nipples." I kept such thoughts to myself. Dr. Keily was now pulling a little here and there on the gauze covering the surgical incisions. He was satisfied to see that there was no drainage or blood and that all was as it should be. While he was checking his surgery, I was checking on my new breasts. My healthy breast had now become smaller and ascended a good inch up on my chest. It looked good and shapely. My implant breast had a nipple and seemed to be the same size as the other. "I truly look double-breasted," I said to myself. I could not help thinking about the ad of the chicken producer, Frank Perdue, showing his T.V. audience, with great pride, the bare breasts of his double-breasted chickens. I felt the same pride at being double-breasted again, even if it was through artificial means, as it was in fact with Mr. Perdue's chickens.

I also kept to myself a most undignified and unsurgical thought even when it gave me a good feeling. The feeling had to do with recognizing that this surgery meant that I could leave behind the preoccupation about my breast. Never again would I have to see if my breasts looked even, if they were at the same height, before meeting a person. I had had an experience of that nature the week before the surgery. My friend Gladys and her children and I had gone together to a resort for the weekend. At night her teenage daughter, who knew nothing about my illness, came to my room to ask something just when I was ready to go to bed and I had taken off my padded brassiere. It was very obvious that my two breasts, the normal one and the expander, were very different. I felt panic that she would notice it and that I would have to explain my illness to her or require of her not to ask questions about something obvious. I did manage to get my brassiere on just before she saw me.

It was the thought of living my life constantly preoccupied about my breasts that had decided me to undertake plastic surgery. A friend had given me an article about a woman who had chosen not to have plastic surgery. She spoke of several episodes when she had felt embarrassed even in front of people who knew her well and who knew about her cancer and her mastectomy. It is the shame about not looking normal, the way one is supposed to look, that is most difficult to overcome. It seems to be a natural human trait to wish to hide that which makes us different from others or ourselves in the past, particularly if that something is an organ we are supposed to have as a matter of course. Even animals seem to share that feeling because most of them hide when wounded, and even in hiding they shield their wounds from the sight of others. There seems to be a universal emotional law that it is shameful to be wounded.

I could feel in myself now the other side of such law. The restoration of my breast, this first sight of my newly implanted breast, gave me a feeling of well-being, of being whole, together, unwounded again. Once more I felt grateful to the surgeon and the surgical team. There was no time to say anything. Dr. Keily had finished his inspection and, now leaving the room, said that I could go whenever I was ready. I said I would be ready the following day.

My friends took over when the hospital released me. I had taken some vacation time for the surgery, and I could go places with them. My friends, Joe and Blondie, took me to their home in a neighboring state. Their 20-year-old son, Thomas, drove me from the hospital to their place. There they pampered me with words, acts, and food, and I felt like a fairy tale princess to whom the best of worlds had been given by a kind fairy godmother. We chatted, watched T.V., walked a little (they live in the country), and hung around the house chatting with whoever was there at the time. Their late adolescent children, who always called me aunt, seemed pleased to have me there, an adult they could relate to who was not a parent. It was a treat for me to have time to spend in long personal chats with children I had known since their infancy. Now they were young men and women, and in listening to them I could see that they were becoming complete persons, my equals in their ability to ponder the wonders of this world.

After a few days I had to report back to the surgeon who was to check the healing of my wounds. All went well with him. He took out the stitches and the blue foam rubber, and now, for the first time, I saw my two breasts directly. I told him how pleased I was with the results of the surgery. He was now fully his old self, voice, smiles, and all. I had forgiven him and was willing to leave the past behind and reestablish full communication with him. He seemed as relieved as I. We chatted about all kinds of matters. He told me that the foam rubber was blue because it was the padding that was used for heart valves and was not itself a surgical material. In the past surgeons had used cotton to exert pressure on skin grafts to facilitate the formation of new blood vessels between the receiving skin and the grafted skin. The results were not too satisfactory. Someone had thought of using foam rubber, and the foam that came with heart valves worked very well after sterilization. I laughed internally at the irony of having my nipples "decorated" with "heart's padding" while I watched him remove the blue circles from my nipples. He placed a yellowish gauze on top of them and then covered my breasts with a light gauze. He said all was going well and that he wanted to see me in two weeks. I was not to lift anything and had to bathe carefully even though it did not matter if some water touched the surgical wound. I said that the nurse in the hospital had suggested

I use a brassiere but that I found it uncomfortable. He said I did not need it and that I should wait until I was ready to wear one. Once more I felt the feeling of relief, of being able to dress for the first time in nine months without having to check if my breasts looked even. I put on my slip and my dress, and I looked just fine.

6

Back to Everyday Life

August 17

On leaving the hospital, I realized that I was not only leaving it and a long episode behind me, but I was beginning a new chapter of my life, now, I hoped, free of cancer, a bit of a bionic woman, half flesh, half plastic, looking normal and trying to get ready to live an ordinary life.

I knew I still had to have periodic check-ups with the oncologist, that I had to deal with the consequences of not having any sex hormones in my body, that I could not avoid the fear of recurrent metastases someday, someplace in my body. I did know that. I also knew that I could not live *for* the cancer I had had. I had to live life as life came to me and keep on making my contribution to this world the best I could. I had to gear myself up to have the courage to live fully, vitally, decisively, creatively. I knew I could use my fears and my past pains as excuses not to participate fully in the act of living. I was also aware that time did count, that my commitments needed a hierarchy of values to rank them. The time was drawing near to move from the exclusive care of my body, to save me, to the care of me, the one who had a body to live in. The care of me meant the care of those I loved and who loved me, the care of those for whom I was responsible, and the tasks in this world that were exclusively mine.

Other matters began to ask for a hearing. I had to take a second look at my financial planning, my will, retirement places, provisions for older age, including provisions in case I did have metastasis. I realized that all these matters required careful consultation and deep thought and that I did not have to do it immediately.

August 18

Now that I was mending, I began to experience a need to look back to reflect on what had happened to me, to transform a moment of life into my personal history.

Many thoughts, feelings, fantasies, even sensations seemed to have been *waiting* for this moment, like well-behaved children who wait for their mother to be free of urgent cares. Now that I seemed ready to attend to them, they all wanted attention at once and seemed unable to wait any longer.

The thought with the deepest and most somber voice sounded like one of Job's consolers, determined to devalue me and place me among those responsible for their fate. It asked, "Woman, what do you have to live for?" It suggested that I did not have the right to live, that is, to live *for* myself because I had no blood relative to live for: no husband, no children, no grandchildren. It implied that it was a selfish and undignified act to try to live *for* myself, for the very pleasure of living itself. It also listed the "fact" that I was not worthwhile enough to have life if I could not pass it on to others. This voice did not attend to any other reality that did not concern a blood relationship to another human being. It had roots in the Old Testament's contemptuous texts of the *sterile* woman; in the New Testament when Jesus curses the unfruitful fig tree; and in the many "oh's" and "ah's" I had heard after my middle 30s each time I said, as simply and humbly as I could, that I had neither husband nor children. It was as though I had not paid my dues to life and now life owed nothing to me, and I did not have the right to ask for a little more life for myself.

My flesh, the very flesh that had now been cut and removed, the flesh of my breast, was the flesh that had not nursed any babies or offered them a soft and tender pillow for their sleepy heads. My accusing voice proclaimed without compassion that there was justice in my being wounded there, where I had committed the sin of not being a mother, that it was right that I was injured in my womanhood because it was in my infertile womanhood that I had offended the fecundity of the earth and interrupted the heavenly regulation of living creatures.

A bass voice repeated with sarcastic irony "Tell me, woman, what do you have to live for?" The voice's pitch dropped even lower when it reached the word "for." In the background I could hear the humming of the young of all living creatures, big and small, echoing in unison "You did not bring us to life, woman. You did not!"

Encircled by the accusing chorus, I felt trapped in my history like a Greek heroine. I felt the weighty pain of lived and unlived past. The pain centered now, like the head of an arrow, in the heart of the heroine pointing poignantly, unrelentingly, to what I had done with my life, a life I could neither undo nor live again.

The voices were the sound of vibrant young flesh. My words could only become the trembling mumblings of an aging woman supplicating for a few more years of life. I had no words to answer.

They persisted: "Woman, what do YOU have to live FOR?"

I threw myself on the ground, as many others had done before me, lying in front of their gods, their queens, their kings, begging for mercy. I said as humbly as I could, "Forgive me, all you living children of all living things. I have not brought forth life. Have mercy on me. Let me live a little more. Let me partake for a while longer of the life I have received from others."

I waited, hoping that somebody would answer me. Nobody did. The ironic bass interrogator and the humming chorus vanished, and I found myself alone in my desolation.

I raised my head slowly in my aloneness. I realized I had hallucinated my guilt and my fears in a moment of frightful awareness. I had realized without knowing—so the voices had informed me—that I felt guilty for wrenching myself away from the grip of a cancerous death that had begun to corrode my breast. I had the guilt of the survivor, of one who had been counted as dead already but who had managed to go on living. I had felt guilty both in the past and now for having let my sexual maturity go to waste without human fruits. I had felt guilty for not having taken at least a child, somebody's else's child, a biological orphan, and for not having brought her or him up. In my 40s, I had seriously considered adopting a child, which is legally possible for a competent single woman.

This old guilt now combined its power with the depth of my sorrow, because in it, in the form of accusation and self-depreciation, I discovered the wish to have had children who would now look after me and care for me in my old age, if I lived that long, or until I died, whenever that might be.

No, that was not the voice of the unknown accuser or of an implacable Greek chorus. It was my feelings of the past and the present that interfered with my right to live a few more years. I realized that if I was to complete in my soul and mind the work of the surgeons and the oncologist, I had to make peace with myself, with my past and with my present, with my errors, my sins, my omissions, and with the vicissitudes of my life. I had to integrate this cancer of my most maternal and tender of organs with my unmotherly life and my unfruitful flesh. I had to accept who I was as I was, including my vigorous actions to escape a cancerous death. I had to assume the responsibility of having kept myself alive.

Just saying the phrase "having kept myself alive" brought to mind the timeless myth of all creatures, where the hero goes to the sacred place to steal life, light, fire, the fruit of knowledge, and enrages the gods of the highest circles, who in their wrath pursue the robber with fierce vengeance.

I realized that my life was not a myth. There was no Zeus to curse me, no devil to burn me forever. I was once more attributing to some higher being feelings of anger and punishment because I felt guilty for fighting so decisively for my own life. How could I, who so determinedly went from one treatment to another, find for myself the right to live fully whatever years I had left? My imaginary accuser's words, "Whom do you have to live for?" seemed to have a great power to make me crumble. I had to start with that little and most wounding of prepositions: for.

What does "for" mean? I ask myself. Does it mean that if I don't live for someone—a husband, a child, a grandchild, someone—I don't have the right to live? It seemed to mean precisely that. Where did such a conviction come from? Was it from my Christian upbringing, always saying that we have to love and serve others? Was it from the endless experiences of people looking at me in a certain way when I said I had neither husband or children? Was it from the common remarks about the death of a parent, "He leaves such a young child" as though parents should not die like anybody else? Was it from the complementary remark, "He did bring up her children; they are now grown up and can take care of themselves," as though there is no need to live beyond the parenting years? Was it from the sad remark made when the member of an elderly couple dies, "He won't live much longer; they could not live without each other," as though one should not live without a spouse? Or perhaps it came from the not so infrequent remark made about very elderly and disabled parents who have just died after years of suffering and invalidism, "It's a relief for her and also for all of us."

Perhaps there were some other sources too: childhood feelings, seemingly long forgotten, that I was not worth bringing into the world because I had failed my parents in their wishes for me. The pitch of their voices when they complained about me and the ways in which I displeased them seemed now related to the tone of the "for" in the imaginary voice.

Finally, I had to have the courage to acknowledge that it was I who was complaining about myself, my disappointment with my lack of "skills" for getting myself a partner and becoming a parent. I found myself daydreaming about imaginary husbands—men I never met. I also reviewed, in the way troops are reviewed, all the men I "could" have married but did not. Before I knew it, I had myself an imaginary past husband and two children. I thought about the names I would have given them. In my imagination I came to have a 29-year-old daughter by the name of Charlotte and a 26-year-old son called Stephen. Suddenly I realized that I was trying to give myself a family in a hurry, to alleviate my guilt and my sorrow all at once.

"No, no," I said, "that is not the way to make peace with yourself and your wifely and motherly failure. You have to face it squarely as it is, as it will be. You are a woman alone who did not marry, did not bring forth children, and you have got to accept it, and [the words now acquired all their meaning] you have to live with 'it.' You have nobody to live 'for.' "

"What does it mean," I asked, "to live 'for' no one? Is it all right to shorten the verbal expression and just 'live,' without the troubling preposition whose persistent demand I simply could not satisfy?"

August 23

I was in this quandary for a while. I had gone with a friend to a resort island on the Atlantic coast to repair my body and soul. There, while

walking in the forest, I kept on asking, what does it mean to "live," just
to live? I realized that from the earliest moments of human awakening
the question had been asked persistently, insistently, and so far no one
seemed to have come up with an answer that could bring peace to the
inner contradictions of the human heart.

Suddenly my childhood Sunday School answer came to mind,
"God made me to know Him [we did not say Her in those days], to
love Him, and to serve Him in this world, and to be happy with Him
for ever in the next." It seemed a pretty neat and fancy answer: simple
as one, two, three—no doubts, no confusion about anything. As a
child I thought it a very good answer because then I was in the habit
of obeying orders from parents and teachers, those who represented
the big God in the sky. Now, however, I had no one to tell me what
to do. I had not even the faintest idea of what "to love and serve
the Lord" meant in my 54th year. Did I have to be like the saints,
like another Mother Teresa, and go and kiss some others who were,
in fact, dying? How could I do such a thing in good conscience when
I had fought so fiercely to keep myself alive? Did I have to do
something heroic, a bit bizarre, as saints have done? Well, truly, I had
no wish to and probably could not carry out such saintly acts without
stopping in the middle to laugh at myself, seeing that I was a complete
fool.

Should I continue doing whatever I had been doing so far, that is,
living a simple, orderly life of seeing patients, reading, writing, going to
supper with friends, puttering around the house, walking the dog,
shopping in the supermarket, watching a few movies and plays, and
then, one day, expiring peacefully out of this earth's atmosphere? Is
this what I wanted life "for"? I heard two voices in me. One seemed
indignant and contemptuous because I was making such a fuss to stay
alive just to do all those most pedestrian things anybody else could do
at least as well as me. It seemed I was asking a lot "for" nothing. The
other voice, softer and timid, came with a feeling that I was cheating.
It said, "I just want to stay alive."

I realized that if I had to present myself to a superior court, I could
not make much of a case. The best I could say was something like,
"Ladies and gentlemen, my patients need me." I could hear their deep
voices saying, "Nonsense, Madam. No one is indispensable. They can
be assigned to one of your competent colleagues." I had nothing to say.
They were right. Before I finished this imaginary dialogue with the
"Supreme Court of the Living," I realized that I had returned through

circuitous roads to the earlier argument of trying to prove that I had something to live "for."

"No," I said, "no, you have nothing to live 'for.' If you want to keep on living, have the courage to say so. Say, 'I want to live' and no more. Have the courage of your wishes," I exhorted myself. "Obviously, you like the act of living itself." This phrase, "Obviously you like the act of living itself," made a sudden and strong impression on me.

"Yes, oh yes," I said, "I do. I really do." This was a new turn of events. I realized how much I liked the stereophonic reality that my senses brought to me every second: the minuscule sounds of life and the big bangs; the dark nights with just one visible star and the bright midday light with its brilliant palette of contrasting colors; the play-fulness of the wind tickling my skin and the mischief of rain falling on me; the weight of my limbs dialoguing with material and human objects; those exchanges of push and pull between me and the world, like a lover's endless embrace. Oh, yes. Oh, yes. I did like life, just as it was – a physical reality of smells and sounds and sights and sensations. Acknowledging that I liked life so much improved my mood at once. "Oh," I said to the Supreme Court, "I think I like to live because life is pleasurable. I like whatever is out there. I mean," I said humbly, "outside myself."

My judges looked at each other and cleared their throats. The oldest spoke gravely, "At last, Madam, you have spoken the truth," and looked at the others, rolling his eyes as though to say what a difficult case I was. I was encouraged by his indications that he was willing to put up with me.

Before I knew it, I was again reviewing troops. This time it was the army of friends. I stood in front of each of them like a platoon sergeant, examining them with scrutinizing eyes. After a while I began to smile because I could not help liking them. At the tail end of the platoon I found the two surgeons, Dr. Robbins and Dr. Keily (whom I had fully forgiven), and the oncologist, Dr. Nagle, and Monique, my nurse. I smiled broadly at them because I could not help liking them too – and quite a lot too.

A lady judge, seeing my excitement, said in a tone not unlike my mother's in the past, "What are you so happy about?"

"My lady of the Supreme Court," I said respectfully and sheepishly, "I like people, too."

"That is fine," she said curtly and looked at the others, rolling her eyes to confirm what a difficult case I was.

Suddenly the Supreme Court vanished, and I discovered that I had
gone out for a walk and was in the middle of the woods on a narrow
foot path. I returned to my senses in a peaceful, almost joyful mood. I
could only hear crickets playing their minuscule harps, birds chirping,
and the soft rustling of leaves and branches caressed by the ocean
breeze. Everything was harmoniously serene. I kept on walking as if in
a timeless dream of unspoken joy. Turning a corner of the path, I saw
to the right of it a large fallen tree trunk. It seemed dead, its dead roots
exposed as a large, circular, dry placenta showing its lifeless surface.

August 23, evening

The dead tree cut a sad and contrasting figure among its neighboring
tall and proud pines, birches, and maples. I sat on a stone to
contemplate the fallen tree and its complex message to me. It had been
a splendid specimen, probably 30 years old if I could judge by the
width of its trunk. I looked at the exposed, dried, vertical roots. Now
they were whitish and terribly dry, like old bones. My eyes followed
the tree trunk for all its length, a good seven or eight feet. The same
whitish grayness covered the surface. At the end, three large branches,
crushed and broken, exposed their amputated stumps, some flat on
the ground, some like lepers' limbs extended upward, mutely imploring. I was feeling very sad for the dead tree. I got up to touch it and sit
on it as though I could console it for its untimely death.

While I walked toward the tree, my eyes suddenly saw a most
unexpected sight. From one side branch I had not seen before, the tree
had produced a majestic, elegant, upright shoot, large, strong and
vigorous, which had harmoniously joined the tree formations in the
woods. It had grown as tall as the others and seemed so normal that if
I were not looking at its foundation, I would not have been able to tell
that that was not a normal tree. I had not seen it before because I had
assumed it was a *normal* tree growing from the ground and encircled by
the dead branches of the tree. I looked in amazement, trying to see
how such a beautiful shoot managed to nourish itself. I reasoned
that the dead trunk was not completely dead. My eyes traveled along
the large trunk until they met the roots again. There I saw that
underneath the fallen stem several roots had arched themselves to

penetrate the ground and had extended themselves in a broad circle underneath the trunk to provide new roots for the shoot.

I sat on the trunk and touched the tree the way a woman caresses her lover who has just returned from combat, with tenderness, admiration, respect, in silence. Tears came to my eyes. This unknown tree in the forest, unconscious of itself, had said in its act of being what I could not say even when I knew it was my wish. The tree had followed its natural law, its compelling need to branch up in search of warm sun, to take its light, its fire, into the tree's life itself. The tree had had the courage to take its portion of fire from the sky to make a living. To be a tree seemed a good enough reason for the creation of a new lease on life, a new shoot after uprooting and massive amputation. I kissed the tree and thanked it for its unintended lesson. I do not know if trees understand kisses, but I had the need to express the gratitude I felt for having found a fellow mutilated being who had made it in its own world.

August 24

The encounter with the tree seemed to settle the matter. I did not have to "live for" anything. I could simply "live" whatever way I could with contortions, distortions, contraptions, and any other props I might need to stay here on earth, warming up under the sun.

It was at this point, when I had the courage to say that I wanted to live for life itself, that I had my next illumination. I realized that there is nothing we can do to bring about life or to keep life except to remove the obstacles that interfere with it. The whole of medicine and surgery are devoted to just that: to join in a life that is already there and help out when there is trouble. Life itself is a given, or if we look at it as Christians, a grace. To say it less theologically, life is "gratis," a gift, free of charge. My discoveries, my encounters with the tree, the illuminations, all converged to lift my mood to a point of serene joy. "Fine," I said (I think I was talking to the Supreme Court of the Living), "as long as I am graced with life, I am going to live it, simply, one hour after the other, doing what I have to do and enjoying the act of living itself."

"Perhaps," said the theologian and the child of the catechism in me, "that is what it means 'to love and serve the Lord': just to love what is there, the grace of life itself." I was careful not to remember half of my catechism answer, "to be happy with Him for ever in the next." I was not ready for higher joys, I reflected apologetically. I had learned just a few hours earlier that I could enjoy the grace of life that my Maker is still giving me, gratis. One cannot learn more than one lesson at a time.

August 27

That night we had a big storm. Gales from the sea swept the land and battered the trees while heavy rain, like a curtain of water, descended from the clouds. The sky celebrated with fireworks of lightning and thunder.

Morning dawned fresh and sunny and full of scents.

I went for a walk in the forest. The rain seemed to have given a magic touch to every tree and every stone. A luminous, moist softness radiated from every flower, every branch, every leaf. Small creatures were singing their canticles, each following a different tune. From the dead leaves came an intoxicating, inebriating smell of fermentation and transformation. The moisture of the night was accelerating the fermentation of lifeless leaves into life-breeding substances. I walked, drunk with the beauty of the early morning. I felt an inner softness, a feeling of peace with myself and the world, with my newly gained conviction that it was good enough to be there, in the community of human beings—like the tree in the forest—carrying out my assigned tasks, simply, faithfully, humbly.

I saw a little flower raising its purple petals no higher than two inches above the ground. They were open, welcoming insects whose sweet drinking from her generous food would make them into messengers of fecundity. I bent over to look at the flower. It was bright purple and made in such proportion and grace that one could suspect it to be the work of the hands of a most delicate artist. At that point another phrase from the New Testament came to my head. It was Jesus saying that not even Solomon in all his glory had worn a purple as magnificent as that of the flowers of the field. The words gave me great joy. Now that I was identifying with small and beautiful creatures that celebrated life by the simple act of being, I felt that the flower had joined the tree from the other day in giving me permission to live for the grace of living itself. The little flower seemed to say, joining her minuscule voice to Jesus preaching in the fields of Galilee (Mt. 6: 28-29), that I too could compete with King Solomon and try my best to make myself beautiful, adorned with whatever purple suited me best.

I found I had instinctively looked at my breasts. I placed my hands on them, cupping them around their shape. I felt grateful, so very grateful to Dr. Keily, who had replaced my lost breast and returned my body to its natural shape. I recalled with a laugh the card my friend had sent just prior to surgery. On the card was a blooming rose tree; inside were two cut-out roses and the caption, "For your new blooming." I felt as though I had "bloomed" a breast, even when all I had done was let Dr. Keily place the implant on me, under my flesh. All the same, it was now mine, and it did look like a nice enough breast, nipple and all.

I looked at the little purple flower once more and felt like winking an eye at her, as though the flower could understand that I felt like her sister in my wish to be beautiful and be dressed in purple. I was in the best of moods, feeling more and more that my ordeal was coming to an end. I kept on walking along the forest path, letting the light and the smells and the canticles inebriate my senses. There were many puddles in the path. I stopped at a large one, and, recalling Narcissus, I leaned over to see my image reflected in the muddy waters. I did not fall in love with myself. I did smile at myself, though, because I was good enough to be. And I winked at myself just to say to that other me on the water surface that I approved of her. She winked back, and we parted.

Now the forest path opened onto a main paved road. I took it for a while to see where it would bring me. While I walked on the road as cars passed here and there, my thoughts returned to everyday life. It was at this point that I thought again of my poor dead friend Elizabeth, who had died of breast cancer two years earlier after a two-year battle with disseminated cancer all over her body. We had been friends since we were nine years old. Unfortunately, we had ended up living in cities very distant from each other and did not see one another more than once every year or two. The friendship, however, kept on growing. We were always frank and open with each other. Five years prior to her death, when we were visiting, I sensed for the first time that Elizabeth had something she did not want to tell me about. I debated between pressuring her and respecting her right to have secrets. I chose respect, saying to myself that in due time she would tell me. I still feel guilty for thinking that her secret could wait. It did not occur to me that it was that she had a lump on her breast. I could have gone with her to the doctor. I could have eased her fears. I simply did not think about it. She was afraid, and when she went to the doctor it was too late. The best modern medicine could offer her was a few years of painful survival.

After her illness became public knowledge, I visited her several times, and we spoke with our usual frankness. She had made peace with her fate and spoke with simple resignation about her premature death. She and her husband had no children. Her husband could not accept her illness and had practically abandoned her to the care of nurses and other relatives. Elizabeth did not dwell on her many and severe pains. She tried to be courageous to the end.

The last time I saw her it was obvious that her days were numbered. My visiting days were limited, and we both knew that we would not see each other again. I said to her the best way I could that if there was something she wished for, I would do anything I could to satisfy her desire. She did not hesitate for a minute. She said, "I want to see the lake again and the mountain and the forest we went to so many times when we were young." Elizabeth was very weak. She could barely walk, and she tired very easily. I knew I could not handle the task alone. I called some mutual friends who had very comfortable cars and who also loved Elizabeth.

My friend Christine and I took Elizabeth to the lake shore where she could contemplate the mountains and see the edge of the forest. She was so exhausted from the trip itself that we had to carry her physically to the chair we had placed at the edge of the lake. She sat there, panting for air and at the same time smiling, inhaling in her labored breathing every scent brought by the light breeze from the lake side. Her eyes seemed to take everything in. Her emaciated, almost cadaverous face beamed with the joy of seeing a landscape we had loved so much in our youth. She sat there quietly, listening, watching, smelling the scents, occasionally touching Christine's hand or mine. Christine left for a moment and returned with a bouquet of wild flowers. Elizabeth smiled joyfully and held them against her nostrils and then looked at each of them, touching their petals. Christine and I had tears in our eyes. We knew Elizabeth was saying good-bye to all the things she loved, including those little flowers of the field. Her sad joy and our sorrow gave the mountains, the lake, the forest, the flowers a new depth of meaning and feeling.

I am still very moved by the memory of that moment. Elizabeth's death a month later affected me deeply. I could not go back for her funeral, and mourning her alone, without the presence of mutual friends was hard. I always have with me the gifts she gave me. A small makeup set for traveling goes with me wherever I go. A picture in my kitchen, a book she gave me speak silently of our lasting friendship.

I realized that it was through the good services of the purple flower that I had thought now about Elizabeth smelling the wild flowers of the lake in her farewell to life. I felt deep pain and sorrow that Elizabeth had not fought for herself, that she had surrendered to her cancer and let it take over her body so fast, so viciously. I wished I could bring her back to life with me and with the purple flower in its morning glory. I felt that I owed it to Elizabeth to keep on fighting the good battle of life. As long as I could celebrate mountains and lakes, forest and flowers, I would celebrate them for her and for me.

My walk had been very long. I turned back and returned to the resort while talking in my head with Elizabeth, my friend who had not fought for her life.

August 28

The evening of that day brought with it unexpected good omens. The resort had prepared a large picnic for all its guests. One of the reasons for the outdoor meal was to get people to talk to each other, to become acquainted as part of the resort's "family." Following the spirit of the celebration, once my plate was filled to the brim I looked around to see people I had not yet met with whom I could sit to eat my dinner. My friend had left the day before, and I was alone. I spotted two couples – obviously retired people – at one of the few picnic tables that still had some empty seats. I asked their permission to join them and sat down. They welcomed me, and we began the small dance of dialogue to figure each other out. It was clear that they had been friends for years. They were all in their late 60s and early 70s. They treated me a little like a youngster. The conversation began to roll with laughter and good humor. Suddenly, someone mentioned cancer, and before I knew it I was witnessing a cancer-survival ritual. They all looked at each other, and then they spoke as in a play, "We all had cancer." "I," said the woman in front of me, "*had* [she accented the word] cancer of the uterus."

"Yes," confirmed her husband, a medical doctor, "she *had* cancer of the uterus. *I* had cancer somewhere [he moved his hand from head to knees]. Well, I mean lung cancer."

"I," said the woman to my right, "*had* breast cancer. A long time ago," and she laughed with pleasure.

Her husband, on my left, echoed, "I had one too, somewhere," and he laughed.

Then almost as a chorus they said, "We *had* cancer," and laughed triumphantly, like soldiers who had been in the worst of battles a long time ago and were now celebrating their glorious victory over the enemy.

I said timidly, feeling silly and hypocritical, "Early detected cancer is no longer the killer it used to be." Obviously the sentence was mainly for my ears, for me, the survivor of a very recent battle with no medals to show for it.

They did not listen to me. They were too satisfied with their achievement, a much better proof than any social words I could throw into their recitation.

We continued eating our barbecue and dessert and chatted convivially. The episode, however, made a big impression on me. It was as though the gods of good omens, or God in person, had sent me these four unlikely angels of good news to give me courage, to invite me to join them in their old age, free of cancer.

To balance this high moment with heavenly messengers, I had a letdown. While I was buying tickets for a boat trip along the coast, the teenaged girl who was selling them watched me walking a bit slowly and using my arms carefully. She looked at me judiciously, with appraising eyes, and said with the innocence of those who have no concern about age, "Are you a senior citizen?" The question jolted me. I could see that her intent was kind, and her eyes were keen. She had seen me laboring to carry my body around while still fatigued and uncomfortable.

I laughed and said truthfully, not to offend her good intent to give me a discount rate, "Ten years to go still." She looked at me again, blushed and said, "I'm sorry. I'm not good at telling people's age." "It is all right," I responded, "At your age it is hard to imagine one can get to be old." I paid my full-price ticket and went on the boat, slowly and carefully so as not to trip on the ropes lying around.

The holiday was coming to an end. The first thing I had to do on Monday after my return on Sunday was to visit with my oncologist. That visit was the transition point between the time for energetic and immediate treatment for cancer – which had already been carried out by my throwing away my diseased breast, taking out the lymph nodes with metastasis, and killing any cancerous cells anywhere in me by chemotherapy – and the time of watchfulness for potential metastasis in my body.

It was a time to look carefully in two directions. I was to look to the past, to place in context what had happened to me, to evaluate the medical significance of it, to understand better the cancer itself and its treatment. It was the time to change the tense of verbs – as my oncologist friend had commanded – saying that I *had had* cancer. I was to make sure that the whole cancer experience was consciously and unconsciously pushed into the past tense. The present tense had to remain available for life and its vicissitudes.

It was also a time to look at the future, to discuss rationally my probabilities for survival and to learn to live normally while remaining watchful. I had to decide about my entire medical care in the future. Would the oncologist accept the responsibility of being my internist, or did I have to return to my internist? Who was going to check the rest of me: flu vaccines, blood chemistry, and other minor problems that I had collected in my years of living?

I liked Dr. Nagle as a person and as a physician. He seemed to be right there with you in a friendly, witty, and yet reserved manner as befits a man who deals with death and life, in that order, all the time. He was outspoken and seemed to take some pleasure in using strong words to say what he thought was right or wrong. In this respect, he reminded me of my pediatrician, Dr. Pellerin, who always spoke clearly and without euphemisms.

That Dr. Nagle was about ten years younger than I pleased me a great deal because it made me feel that I would have him for a long time. In my selfishness I calculated that he would not retire until I was 75 years old! I was giving myself a 20-year survival time!

I prepared for my meeting with Dr. Nagle as an accountant prepares taxes: I made a very long list of questions and points to make sure that nothing that needed to be discussed would go unnoticed.

September 2

Dr. Nagle and I had our visit together. He saw me in the waiting room and after checking that I was first on the patient's list, he made one of his understated comical gestures with his eyebrows and fingers, indicating that I should wait inside the office. After ten minutes he came in, looked at me to check my emotional level, and said hello in a friendly and neutral manner. It was clear that he was waiting for me to give the hum for the emotional tone of our encounter. I felt totally comfortable with him. I knew I could express my thoughts and feelings. I went directly to what was essential for me at that point: how to go on living, making sense of myself and having the courage to live the life I had fought to keep with his help. I told him that I had not yet made peace with myself, that the psychological work was the medical work now. I told him how afraid I was of the future without a family and how terribly sad it was that my distant relatives and I could not communicate with each other, and that it was not only on account of the distance. There were other, unseen and unnamed, deeper, and more confusing family pains, resentments, feelings of betrayal—the usual family tragedies in which so much of life and good will is wasted on contradictory expectations. We talked about my sister, my mother, my brother, and our entanglements in the web of wished-for love as an eternal spring of pained hope and convoluted resentments. I talked about not having a family of my own.

Dr. Nagle listened carefully, asking a question here and there. He did not console me. He did not minimize my predicament. He simply indicated he understood that it was a predicament and that I had to find peace within myself in dealing with my circumstances and my future. I repeated that I knew I was not yet ready to do that but that I was doing as much as I could to complete his medical treatment while struggling with my problems in life and in living. He punctuated the end of this part of the visit with one of his understated jokes. We both laughed. Then he gave me a gown (one of those white ones with little blue flowers), dashed out of the room to let me change, and returned in a few minutes to examine me.

He went over my body with fingers that knew how to search for the abnormal. He concentrated on his work, talking only to tell me to breathe or what to do. It pleased me that he was immersed in the task of checking my body. Finally he said, "You are very well." His voice sounded pleased, like that of a man who has found a good crop in his vegetable garden. His work had borne fruit.

Then he said that I looked rested, and it seemed to him I had lost some of the weight I had gained before. I laughed, pointing to my midriff. "These rolls [I held the folds of my skin in between my fingers] are not mine."

He retorted, "One of these days you will have your own Rolls."

I did not waste any time in replying, "A Royce is not something I think I'll have." We both feigned seriousness, enjoying the silliness of our words.

He sat down and pointed to the questions in my notebook. "What do you have in your notebook?"

We covered everything: his understanding of my cancer, the prognosis, the good omen that I had tolerated the treatment so well. We discussed my blood chemistry, the future checkups, flu vaccines, vigilance for the possible cancers in my body. He answered my questions thoughtfully, in a matter of fact way, with extended and clear explanations.

Then he told me about the follow up, at first every three months, then every six, then every year. At that point we fell silent. We knew what we were both thinking: would I have metastasis, or would I be one of those lucky ones who have truly eradicated the cancer and never have it again? I thought to myself, "Will I join the choir of my fellow vacationers chanting, 'I had cancer a long time ago' "? Dr. Nagle got up and told me to have my blood drawn. We bid each other farewell until the next visit.

That visit to Dr. Nagle was a milestone. It signified the cease fire in the battle between breast cancer and me. For the time being I could say without doubt, "I *had* cancer." Now there were no more shots, no more strategic moves, no persecution of the enemy. The white flag was hoisted to signal the beginning of peace.

I felt like a soldier in the trenches after the deafening sound of cannon and the total absorption with the battle has come to an end. A sudden great silence and a restless quiet overtake the idle fighter. There is nothing to do; there is no enemy; there is nothing to hear; all is silent. There are no orders, no tasks, no urgent mission. The fierce combatant is off duty. The soldier is now a person, a living person among corpses and weapons in the wasteland land of the battlefield.

My battle was over. The past was past. Now I had to take myself,

wounded, healed, scarred, marked in my flesh forever, to the marketplace of everyday life. I had to live like everybody else.

I discovered that reentry to the world I had left to join the frenetic
battle against cancer was not easier than returning home after having
been in the front. I wished I could erase the whole ten months of my
ordeal, truly forget about it, make believe it never happened to *me*. I
wished in my foolishness that I could be like those who go into a fugue
state and cannot remember what they have done for weeks or even for
years. But I could not forget. All I could do was to accept what had
happened to me and make it a part of my life, my past, my present,
and, most specifically, my future, my ambivalently wanted future. I
wanted more life. I feared to get involved again, to be enticed by life,
like a child immersed in play, and then be suddenly disrupted by
mestastatic cancer. I was becoming afraid of letting the pleasure of life
seduce me into a passion for something that could brook no disruptions.

I needed, like soldiers who return from the front, a ritual of passage,
a ceremony to demonstrate the line between the war past and the
present everyday life.

September 3

My feelings were contradictory. I was elated and relieved. I was sad
and exhausted. I walked around a bit disoriented as though I had to
recognize, to rediscover, what had been familiar to me.

I got home from the visit to the oncologist and proceeded to change
my clothes. I took off everything and stood in front of the mirror,
naked, contemplating the body returned from the war. The day before
the mastectomy I had done the same. I had looked at my body with its
two symmetrical and well-formed breasts for the last time. Caressing
my diseased breast, I had thanked it for serving me well and apologized
to it for having to wrench it out of my body. Now the geography of my
chest showed the marks of battle. My breasts were both smaller. The
healthy one had been reduced in size to match the "implant" breast.
The healthy one showed its pride in looking shapely, even if red and
still swollen from the plastic surgery. It was wounded by several
incisions and was in the process of healing. One incision was located
just under the fold between chest and breast. Another, departing from

the middle of the breast's base, ended around the nipple encircling it. They both had the redness of injured flesh in the process of healing.

The other, my "bionic" breast, had a nipple and areola made by the plastic surgeon out of the skin he had taken from the healthy breast. It had no nerves and no sensation. I touched it while remembering the richness of dialogue my old nipple used to have. My finger found a little button that did not respond. The shape of the breast was geometrically pretty close to my other breast. However, I could see the pectoral muscle that held the implant, flattening it out during its unavoidable contractions to move my arm. The famous "port" of the expander had left its imprint in my body. Under my "bionic" breast there was a sort of elongated vertical lump, starting from an incision at the level of the fold between breast and chest. I touched it. It was hard, as though the body had created a capsule of tissue for the now-removed "port." There were no other wounds in that breast. The skin was smooth and shiny. At the extreme corner, under the armpit, there was a deep cavity, the result of the mastectomy and the removal of lymph nodes. The plastic surgeon could not fix it. If I lifted my arm, anyone could see that I had been wounded and had lost some of my flesh. I looked at myself now, globally, as one looks at a landscape. I remembered the desolate look of a totally flat chest on the mastectomy side after the surgery. I had seen my ribs under the skin, crossed diagonally by the red mastectomy wound. Now the landscape had changed. The desert had grown a mound under my skin, and it had a great similarity to a breast. A good artist, however, or any good observer for that matter, could tell in the blink of an eye that that was not the work of nature but of human hands.

I stared at myself with a fierce determination to accept, truly accept, that from now on this was my postwar body. Sad as I might feel about my wounds, this was, "bionic" or not, MY BODY, my home for living. To signal that I meant what I said, I caressed my two breasts with both hands to indicate that I was not going to discriminate between nature and implant, between my flesh and my artifact. I welcomed them with their new looks as a mother welcomes her maimed children who return from war.

I got dressed without a brassiere, which I was not to use for three months, until all the wounds were completely healed. The dressed me showed that I had two breasts slightly uneven in size. I knew that many women are naturally uneven. I had not been one of them. Only

I and those who knew me intimately would notice the difference. For the world at large, I was again a *bi-breasted* woman.

I went for a walk to relax and enjoy the afternoon and to let myself be among all other creatures.

While walking I noticed that I was becoming a bit weird. I was behaving like a lecherous man, ogling women's breasts, squinting my eyes to measure their size, evenness, shape, and firmness. I realized, not without a certain horror, that for a good 10 or 15 minutes I had undressed in my mind every woman who had crossed my path.

September 4 [continuation of previous entry]

It was the envy of a miser. I coveted other women's naturally healthy breasts. In my malice I also wanted to "see" that they too were a bit defective. I was wishing that they had "bad" breasts like me, so that we could all be equals in our lowest common breast denominator.

While busy sizing women's breasts, my mind lost no time in developing a moderate case of paranoia. I felt that "they"—all of "them," men, women and children and maybe even dogs—were all staring at my breasts and shaking their heads, "knowing" that I had abnormal breasts. I caught myself, and, pointing my psychiatric finger at myself, I admonished as gently as I could, "You are projecting. It is you who are ogling them."

I had not yet improved from this syndrome during my first public walk in my neighborhood after the plastic surgery when I discovered another symptom I had forgotten I had. I was walking past my hairdresser's shop. I had not seen him in a year. I had not been able to get myself to deal with my hair. It had not fallen out as expected, and I had developed a superstitious feeling that if I cut it, something ominous would happen. It was now very long, and I had to make a decision because it was looking a bit wild. I could not decide whether to cut it in the old way—then my extra pounds would be more obvious—or to get a new style. I was stuck in the middle, not able even to think of calling my hairdresser. I was afraid he would detect the truth. He knew a lot about hair, and I feared he would notice something, ask me questions, and that it would be very hard for me not to be truthful to a man who had always been kind to me. So I passed by the shop, like a coward, unable to face my hair dresser.

I returned home in low spirits, overwhelmed by the feelings evoked by my official reentry into the world of the living. I felt the weight of the world of life on my shoulders, the need to carry myself, maimed body and fearful soul, day after day and night after night, attending to the chores of life, my obligations, my commitments. Life felt to me like an endless conveyor belt passing in front of me with the things I had to do without delay. My mood grew gloomier. My spirit left me. In my dark hour, life did not seem worth the effort. Was this what I had fought to keep? Why didn't I let myself die? What was I going to do now, stuck as I was with the endless task of living each day from beginning to end with its demands for food, for rest, for relatedness, for a bit of affection and love, and for a pinch of prestige and glory; living each day with its obligations to others, its bills, its phone calls, the cat to feed, the dog to walk, friends to call, plants to water, correspondence to read, taxes, banks, town hall, and inspectors to attend to? The conveyor belt, that endless ribbon of life, went on and on. The burden was on my shoulders. My knees buckled. My will gave out, and I wished for the first time in my life that I could die a total, final, absolute death. I did not mean a Christian death, with a good God welcoming me and an eternity like another conveyor belt, a sort of "joyful" obligation to sing "Glory, Hallelujah." I felt the eternal fatigue of "having" to sing to the Lord. No, I wanted a rest, an undisturbable rest. I wanted to close my eyes, feeling that it was the last time I "*had*" to do something. I wanted not to be, not to think, not to feel the immense burden of consciousness. I understood now some of my suicidal patients wishing that death would bring them a restful place for their exhausted souls.

I too was exhausted and needed a resting place. Now that the war was over, the combat was raging within me, weakened as I was by actual physical fatigue and an immense psychic fatigue. The accumulated effort to remain courageous for ten months had now collapsed under the release of its own force, and I had collapsed together with it. I was now a fragile, frightened, physically weak middle-aged woman who was alone and who wanted to take a nap before reentering life's main road.

September 6

I did not want to be a woman alone. I do not mean I was without faithful friends. I did have them. But I wanted something more. I

wanted the intimacy of a shared, very personal relationship, a dialogue of souls and bodies with a man who was willing to share my fear
of life, my wish for life, my wanting to commit myself to life again.

I knew I was dreaming and wishing like a fool. I had read in
Newsweek some time ago that any woman over 35 was more likely to
die in a terrorist attack than to find a male partner. I could see that the
statistics would drop below the line if one considered a professional
woman in her 50s, full of stitches and without hormones. I grew very
sad and despondent, prone to hysterical tearfulness, like an old maid
of unliberated Victorian days.

I recalled the story of Boya, the world's finest Chinese zither player
according to Han's legends. His tale was one of deep friendship and
sorrow. He had a friend, Zhong Ziqui, who was his audience. He
would listen to Boya's playing on the zither and would sigh, transported in his ecstasy to the Tai mountains. "How wonderful is the
music!" he would exclaim, "It is as imposing as the Tai mountains!"
One day Ziqui died. Boya had lost his soul mate, the only one worthy
of his music. In his sorrow he broke his zither, cut the strings, and
never played again.

I was like Boya. I did not want to play the music of life without a
Ziqui, a soul mate attuned to its melody, a true sharer of deep
harmonies. Like Boya, struck by sorrow, I wanted to destroy my
musical instrument and enter into a great undisturbed silence.

That was the night of my soul after the battle was over. It was as
long as nights are long—in their seven hours—for those who are in
pain, in waiting, in labor's pain.

Dawn came upon me, slowly and not without effort. It left the field
humid with the dew of my tears and cold with the morning chill of an
unknown new day.

The new day shone on me unrequested. The others—neighbors,
friends, acquaintances, colleagues, patients, cleaning woman, mailman, tax collector—all got out of their beds too, went out of their
homes, and busied themselves. They took me for granted and drafted
me into their business as a matter of course. Even my cat demanded
that we play together, and my dog insisted on walking. It seemed that
life could not go on without me, even if I did not feel like going on. I
found myself encircled in the business of everyday affairs. Life and
loving people had pushed me back, in spite of my wishes. That was my
external life. In my heart I had not settled the matter.

September 8

A friend of mine, Harry, a good and broad minded Buddhist scholar, hearing me and my wishes said, "You are suffering from Buddha's temptation."

"What is that?" I asked. He said that after Buddha had attained the highest insight, while sitting under the fig tree on the shore of the Neranjara River, he was tempted by Mara, the evil one. Buddha's temptation, he said, was to *enter* Nirvana—where there is neither suffering nor desire—and stay there forever.

The Holy One—like me—wanted to enter the eternal calm of Nirvana. He did not want to go around preaching the doctrine because he thought, "It will bring me weariness and labor."

The version of the Mahavagga book, Harry instructed me, says that the highest Brahma of the Brahma heaven, Brahma Sahampati, appeared to the Holy One and begged and supplicated him to go and preach the doctrine so other creatures could experience Buddha's illumination.

The Holy One resisted the first two supplications of the highest Brahma. The third time "having heard Brahma's exhortations [he was] seized with compassion for living creatures" and "gazed with a Buddha's eye over the world." He saw human beings wrestling with their condition and "he saw many among them who lived in fear of the coming life and of sin."

Moved by compassion, the Holy One renounced *entering* Nirvana for the sake of his fellow humans.

He responded to Brahma Sahampati:

For all be opened the portals of eternity,
Let him with ears hear the word with faith.
Afraid of toil, I kept from men
the bright and noble word, O Brahma.

Once Buddha had made his promise, the highest Brahma bowed to the Holy One and vanished from sight.

"Then," Harry continued, "one of the books of Mahayana, *Sāntideva*, reveals the vow of the Bodhisattva":

And I take upon myself the burden of all sufferings. I am resolved to do so. I bear them . I turn not back. I do not flee. I quake not, neither do

I tremble. I fear not. I yield not, nor do I hesitate. And why? Because I must take upon me the burden of all beings. *It is not my free will.* The deliverance of all beings is my solemn vow.

Even when I felt very despondent, I was greatly consoled by learning that 2,600 years ago, a man in India, who did not have cancer or other known physical illness, but the ordinary pains of life, had wanted to enter Nirvana all by himself. The triple supplications of the highest Brahma were needed for him to be drafted against his will to preach the doctrine to humankind. He too had had a dark night, a temptation, and a wish to quit.

I was much delighted—and only half consoled—by Harry's learned instruction and by his good efforts to show me that I was hurting from the deep-seated pains of being a human being, scared of toil and suffering.

The story caught my fancy. I was secretly pleased that I had such an illustrious companion. It felt most fulfilling to say, "Buddha and I want to enter Nirvana *now*." Harry laughed and, letting his pragmatic side come to the fore, said with sympathetic malice, "Why don't you try to enter Nirvana *now*?"

I had to concede that I was going against my will because no matter how much I wanted to enter Nirvana, Nirvana was nowhere to be found. So I too, like the Holy One, had to make a vow to stay with all creatures. The problem was to stay with love and compassion as he did and not like a bitter old hag. A bit of grace and clean-heartedness was called for.

Now that I was only half despondent I made a mistake. Another friend came to visit, a learned Lutheran friend, Cornelia, who complemented the practice of internal medicine and bringing up three children with dedication to the understanding of her Christian commitment. I told her I was despondent and how Harry's Buddha story had served me well. She did not know Harry, but in her Lutheran zeal (she is as passionate as Martin Luther himself) she felt compelled to balance my Buddhist consolation with her Christian faith. I was sure she felt Harry to be a competitor in the mission of bringing me to my senses. Before I knew it I was hearing something that could be called a kind, first rate, private sermon without a pulpit.

She proceeded to tell me that Christ's temptation throughout his public life was a constant invitation to take himself for granted, rejoice in the fact that he was the Messiah, perform splendid miracles, and escape the terrible suffering and death that awaited him. She reminded me – her fellow Christian – that St. Luke in his Gospel (4:13) talks vividly about Christ's temptations and that St. John's Gospel (12:27) describes the reluctance of Jesus to go to his suffering and how this other Holy One prayed, "Father, save me from this hour." Cornelia's eloquence reached its highest point when she said that we all – Buddha, Christ, she and I and all others – are invited into the pain of life as our participation in the process of universal redemption. She conceded generously that even Buddha had understood that very well, if he had made the vow Harry said he had made. Cornelia ended the sermon by inviting me to accept my suffering with compassion for the suffering of all other people and with sympathy of heart as a follower of the man who was acquainted with grief. I responded meekly and mischievously – I did not want to give in – with a scriptural citation: "The spirit is ready, but the flesh is weak."

Cornelia was not about to let me swim in my sea of sorrow. Following the example of Brahma Sahampati, she made her exhortation twice and then a third time. She said, "Madeleine, you are not alone in your fear, your fatigue and suffering. The whole world is with you. There is so much suffering, so much tragedy in the world. If each of us bears her share patiently and gently, then we do not add sorrow to pain. There will be better days for you. Just be patient and live one day, one hour at a time. Try to enjoy the little things that come along your way. You have only this life to live. You are living it now. Don't let your pain transform the life you have today into wasted time. There is always time to die, always time to retreat. Today is the only time we have to be ourselves, to be with others, with the world, with all things that share with us their small breath of life." She had talked tenderly to me, measuring each word she said. I felt her affection and her eagerness to see me pull out of my wish for retreat.

Listening to her, I experienced as many contradictory feelings as one can have in a minute. I knew she was right. I both did and did not want to be stubborn. I was full of hesitation. I was afraid. I was flattered that Harry and Cornelia had brought in the two greatest beings in history as their witnesses to console me. I was moved by their tender love. I was secretly complacent, like a stubborn child who enjoys seeing his parents despair if she doesn't move. It was the pleasure of the hidden power of the frightened and stubborn little one over the impotent grown ups: Harry, Cornelia, and their numerous unnamed assistants called my friends. Not without shame did I notice that I liked my sorrow. It made me feel entitled to exercise without guilt a total act of civil disobedience toward life: a life strike.

I thanked Cornelia for her fervent exhortation and, touching her hand, I said, "Be patient with me. I'll come around. Let me take my time. I did hear you. You are right. Wait for my flesh to catch up with my spirit. I am confused. I don't know what I need. I don't know what I want. I don't even know what I fear. I need time and your patience." Then—not without pleasure—I said, "Harry and his Buddha would have to wait exactly the same amount of time as you and *your* (I was at the height of my malice) Jesus."

She smiled and said softly (ignoring my malice), "I know. Just remember that we [she meant many friends] care about you. You can count on us."

I knew I could, and I felt a bit guilty, just a little bit, for being mean to her. "I know," I said, and I meant it.

Then, before I knew it, we were talking as usual in an animated way about all kinds of things and people and medicine and the nation and the children as we had always done.

By the time Cornelia left, my heart had warmed up. I realized that, without knowing it, I had reentered the world of human beings and had forgotten for an hour or so about my Nirvana. So it was from now on. Unlike Buddha, I made no vow to Brahma that I would bring the word to all creatures. Unlike Jesus, I did not have the courage to say in one breath, "Let your will be done" because he loved the Father and His brethren. I felt too little, too scared, too exhausted. I rejoined my fellow creatures in little steps, carried away by the everyday invitation of my friends and the little temptations of life: a good meal, a beautiful flower, laughter, a good book, interesting news. Radio and television seemed to have plotted against me, tempting me at the two horns of my dilemma. They persisted in offering every imaginable contraption and article from cereal to tractors, passing through mattresses, tooth paste, insurance and cars to make me the happiest, most carefree, most beautiful, best smiling person in the country. They assured me that happiness was in the eating of my cereal or in the driving of a red convertible. Happiness was just at the tip of my fingers.

With equal insistence, the two evil plotters kept on giving the "news." "Seven murdered in supermarket by Vietnam veteran." "An earthquake in Mexico–many dead and homeless." "473 children infected with AIDS." "20,000 soldiers killed in Iran." "Today is the anniversary of the explosion of the space shuttle in front of the whole world." "Famine in Ethiopia." "Harsh words between Reagan and Gorbachev." "Nicaraguan rebels want more money." "Ten Salvadorans died of suffocation trying to immigrate illegally into the U.S.A." "The President wanted more money for his ADI. 'It could destroy in a few seconds,' he said, 'some atomic weapons aimed at banishing the U.S.A. from the world's surface.'"

It was through this modern, airborne, acoustical, and visual accumulation of radio and T.V. waves that little by little I had my *enlightenment.* I was hearing and seeing the endless and foolish suffering that we impose upon each other, the hatred of nations and individuals, the tragedy of contagious illness, the horror of murderous madness, the terrifying power of a blind nature. This must have been the material and spiritual suffering that so moved the hearts of Buddha and Christ. "This," I said in my now sober and mature hour, "this is our world: suffering, confusing meanings, tragedy, and a driving need for love, fellowship, and happiness."

"This," I said as simply as I could, this time with humility, "this is the world to which I belong. I should take my place in it. I should accept my share of suffering. I should not hide my longings for happiness." Suddenly I heard myself and laughed at my great solemnity. I was talking as though I were big, as big as Buddha or Christ.

To balance my solemnity and remind myself of my size, I made a civilized commitment to radio and television: I'd try to be "happy" with my cereal, to be beautiful with the creams, to enjoy my car, to think myself the happiest person in the world, and to feel as protected as anyone could be, because Caretakers No Slumber Insurance Co. had insured all of my properties.

After I made these vows to Life and to life (radio–T.V.) I fell peacefully asleep and dreamed that I was canoeing with some friends down a calm little mountain river.

September 13

The day after my solemn attempt at reconciliation with Life and life, I had an appointment with the plastic surgeon to check the result of his sculpting work on my chest. Dr. Keily was in his best mood. I had a dream about him. I dreamed that my family and I, a child of seven, arrived at a public park where a large picnic was being held. We drove a very old, beat up car from the 30s; it was black with yellowish blotches of vanished paint, the result of encounters with hard objects, the car's life wounds. The car was a mixture of my uncle's car in my childhood – a Chevrolet with a rumble seat, a trunk that opened as a seat – and a car in a movie I had just seen. When the car stopped, Dr. Keily, who was walking in the direction of the picnic tables, turned around, winked, and grinned, gesturing an invitation for me to join him in the fun. The image was a visual illustration of his most playful way of saying the word "fun" and his five-year-old disposition to play the responsible job of making little mounds of flesh – transformed mud pies – on women's chests.

In the dream I loved him for his genuinely welcoming gesture. He was inviting me to join in the party of life, which he seemed to enjoy himself.

During my actual visit, we chatted a little. I told him about my minor discomforts. He listened and reassured me that all was fine. After the examination, he took out a few stitches with a gentle hand. I was amazed to see how much surgical thread could be hidden within the little button of a reconstructed nipple. When the surgical procedures were finished, Dr. Keily leaned against the wall of the small office (I was sitting on a very high stretcher facing him at his eye level) and fixed his gaze on my breasts. I could see that he had entered the dreamland of surgery and that his eyes and brain were palpating, sensing the tissues, going to the depths of my flesh, pondering, perhaps repeating moments of the surgery. After a long period of totally concentrated thinking about what was under my skin, his eyes focused on the surface of my breasts and the nipples. They darted to the right, to the left, to the right again, back to the left. Finally a broad grin came upon his face, and, looking first at his nurse then at me, he said with proud satisfaction, "It looks pretty good to me. What do you think?"

I said that it looked pretty good to me too. I told him how grateful I was that I could dress normally and did not have to be concerned with how I looked. I thanked him for convincing me that it was best for me to have plastic surgery. "Well," he said calmly, speaking as the competent, sober evaluator of a factual surgical reality, "your breasts do look symmetrical enough, and the implant on your right breast will become softer and more shapely in a few months. It takes from three to six months for it to soften and be closer to a natural breast." "However," he said with a slightly lower pitch, "your right breast will not have the full shape, the coming forward of your left breast. It will not be noticeable when you are able to wear a brassiere." His voice dropped another octave. "Unfortunately, you'll never have sensation in your nipple. It has no nerves."

I felt that he felt for me and my predicament, and I enjoyed the consolation offered by his changing voice, like a child being soothed by her parent's caring voice. To help my sadness, I touched the sensationless nipple with my left index finger and said to him and to myself, "I know, poor little thing (I was talking to my nipple), you can just do one thing: be a little button there where a button should be."

He said nothing and gave me time to handle myself. Then he asked me if I had any questions. I wanted to know if I could swim. (I had 13 pounds to lose.) He said yes, as much as I wanted. I asked what restrictions I had in the use of my arm. He said that I had none. I laughed, and thinking I had to fix a few odds and ends in my house that needed some carpentry skills, I said to myself, "So I can be a carpenter." He looked at me, not knowing whether I was serious or crazy. He solved the question by washing his hands. While drying them, he asked how I was feeling in general. I said that I was much better and that now that I was feeling restored and with apparently normal breasts, I was feeling like a bionic woman, half flesh, half synthetic.

He turned around and laughed openly, wasting no time in saying to the nurse and to me, "She is a very expensive woman." He again entered his surgical private world and after making some private calculations said that if my schedule permitted he wanted to see me in three weeks to a month. We discussed what he wanted to check: some of the stitches in my left breast. There was a problem with the scheduling. After some discussion we finally agreed that the best thing was for me to call him in two weeks and then decide what to do.

I left in a great mood. He was again the man I had met the first few times: honest, thoughtful, playful, competent. There is nothing so reassuring to a patient as to feel that the physician is a person of real integrity, capable of sober compassion and whose clinical judgment prevails over any other consideration. I reexperienced the feeling I had had in my dream about him. Dr. Keily, by his manner and his actions, had extended me an easy-to-accept invitation to the party of life. He indicated, without saying it, that I could go as I was now: wounded, healed, and scarred.

Following his hint, I decided while walking to my car that I would go to a store specializing in clothes and prosthesis for mastectomy patients and buy myself a "sexy" bathing suit. I was determined to go swimming as soon as possible. I could not use my old bathing suit because I had the deep well under my armpit, and I needed to cover it so as not to reveal my surgical history.

That was my lucky day. The store had a sale and after a goodly amount of searching, trying one and another bathing suit, I found one that fit me perfectly without revealing any of my anatomical secrets. The suits are purposely made to reach very high under the arm, and they have a well-formed brassiere. The brassiere covers whatever unevenness there is in the breast. Seeing myself in the full-length mirror, appearing like a normal, plump, middle-aged woman wearing a bathing suit, gave me as good a feeling as if I had just been acclaimed Miss Universe. My vanity returned in the blinking of an eye, and I found myself imagining how good I would look with ten pounds less. I was enjoying the double pleasure of having a new garment and paying for it at a sale price. A bargain is a bargain!

The following day I ran out of the office to go swimming. The paranoid person of my days of ogling my neighbor's breasts returned at once when I realized that other women could see me changing or showering because the stalls had no curtains and everybody was very casual about showing their naked bodies.

It was once more time for the sensible person to confront the suspicious paranoid. I found, not without a struggle, a Solomonic solution to my dilemma. "They" could look at my behind as much as they wanted. The front of me was reserved for the eyeless wall of the shower stall, and not even under police orders would I be willing to turn around. That did it. I marched toward the shower wrapped in my towel and unwrapped myself within the stall according to the new rule. I saw from the corner of my eye that most women did the same — a detail I had never noticed before. This was how I found out that I was statistically normal as far as showering was concerned. That hump was over.

The next one was to see how the suit would hold its shape once wet. It did. Reassured that no one but me knew that I had something to hide, I felt elated, like a fish in water. I had little stamina to make a big display of my swimming abilities; I just let my body glide in the warm water, feeling the full pleasure of being enwrapped in so tender a creature, "chaste sister water," as St. Francis had called it.

It had been a long time since I had felt a true bodily pleasure, a harmonious well-being between me and myself, me and the world. While I floated on my back on the pool, a great joy came upon me. I had a wish to dance, to sing, to celebrate the return of the zest for life to my body.

I went to the shallow part of the pool and, fantasizing that people would think I was doing some weird aquatic aerobics, I invented a little water dance, humming softly a secret simple tune of my younger days.

At the end of the day, I looked back at what joys and travails it had brought me, and I said quietly that it had been a good day, like one of those evenings at the time of creation when God saw that what he had brought to life was good and he liked it.

That night I slept well and dreamed that a dark bird had flown away. I could see it getting smaller on the horizon while my cat, Michou, sitting on the window sill, contemplated the bird's flight with wide reflective eyes. The front doorbell rang in the dream. It was the mailman, who had a registered letter from a friend abroad. The mailman said, "I hope it is good news." The alarm woke me up before I could read the letter.

September 27

It was now time to catch up with all the postponed everyday obligations that had had to be ignored during those long months of constant medical visits and physical exhaustions. It was time also to attend to other parts of me that did not clamor for attention. I had to see my ophthalmologist to check my glasses. I was reading very far away from the text, and I needed new glasses. My dentist had sent me a reminder that I was long overdue for a checkup. My cat needed her vaccinations. The plumber had to be called to fix a small leak. I had a pile of letters to answer. My plants needed trimming, transplanting, repotting, and fertilization. My kitchen's extra supplies for emergencies were depleted and had to be restocked. Many of my shoes needed new heels. Several of my clothes were long overdue for a visit to the cleaners, and there were other things I cannot recall. The cogwheels of daily little events were beginning their circular movement again. I had, like a factory worker, to be ready to do my job when the conveyor belt presented the task to me.

Thinking that if I was going to get moving I might as well see what I was doing, I started with the ophthalmologist. As soon as I got to the appointment I felt the pangs of doubt and worry. I had to tell him about my cancer. I did not want to. I knew it would be a brief report in which I had to condense 11 months of great pain into a sober informative sentence. I feared his reaction and mine. It was this first move outside the immediate realm of cancer that made me aware that I was extremely reluctant to talk about it with people who had not known my ordeal. A feeling of "it is none of your business" came upon me as though a violation of my soul would follow the disclosure of what had happened to me.

I found myself doing something I did only in moments of great anxiety. I was rehearsing every possible way of starting my cancer report, trying to imagine the impact the words would have on Dr. Stonewell. I could feel that all of me resisted saying any of the sentences. I even considered some way of manipulating the consultation to avoid telling him anything. I imagined his asking me how I had been in these last two years. He knew about some minor medical problems I had had and, as a good clinician, he always asked careful questions about them. I would use an elliptic answer like, "My eyes have not given me any trouble," making believe that I had only eyes to talk about. Worse thoughts came to me. What about a lie. "Fine, Dr. Stonewell, everything is fine!" Then I imagined his saying something like, "There is something unusual in your retina. Did you have chemotherapy?" No, there was no way out. I felt the fear of a child who has stolen cookies and is afraid of saying she has not because there may still be some crumbs in the corners of her mouth. Dr. Stonewell, I feared, would find me out. I had to tell him. Maybe he would be in a great hurry and would ask no questions. I knew, though, that he would take the time, regardless of what else he had to do. There was no escape. I had to tell *if* I did go. Maybe I would not go. Finally I gritted my teeth and told myself that I had to go and let things happen as they would.

I tried to understand my reluctance. After some reflection, I realized that I was heir to a very long tradition of humankind. There have always been horrifying illnesses, capable of awakening tremendous fear, disgust, horror. They have changed in the course of time, along with the progress of the therapeutic results of medical efforts. In biblical times and until quite recently, leprosy was the horror of horrors. In the last century and for a good part of our century it was tuberculosis. Nowadays cancer had taken the first place until AIDS, with its uncontainable march toward a certain death, relegated cancer to second place.

I did not want to become, in the minds of people, the name of my illness, as so many unfortunate men and women in the past had been. I did not want to be first a leper and then me. I did not want to be the chill in my neighbor's spirit: "She has cancer." I wanted to be first and have cancer be a minor qualifier of me. I realized now – in my sober mood – that I had no power over this matter, that each person would react according to her or his own fears and experiences in the past, that some would feel the horror of my having cancer and would avoid me or treat me differently as a way of magically avoiding IT. Some would try not to inform themselves about my having IT, and some others would put it into the context of "me" and of the nature of human life: a mortal adventure. So I went at the appointed time to see Dr. Stonewell. I was sitting on the high ophthalmological chair after the optometrist, a young woman of gloomy mood, made me read the chart with assorted glasses.

Dr. Stonewell, a short, timid, soft-spoken man, came in, shook hands, and said, while looking at me with scrutinizing eyes, "How have you been?" He had my chart in his hand, and it was obvious he had reviewed what had to be checked. I felt his gaze upon me, and I said, avoiding his eyes, "Not well. I had breast cancer, infiltrating, and two metastatic lymph nodes. I had a mastectomy and plastic surgery and also a full course of chemotherapy." I said it all in one breath, like a child reciting an incantation or a lesson she did not like to learn.

He said calmly, "That is not a good thing to have," and then quietly, as a matter of course, Dr. Stonewell asked about details of diagnosis, treatment, and prognosis. There was compassion and respect – no horror – in his dialogue with me. He examined me and told me triumphantly that my eyes were in *perfect* shape and that my retinas showed no signs of arteriosclerosis. "Your eyes are *perfect*," he said very emphatically, as though he wanted me to know that some part of me was as perfect as it could be imagined. I felt very pleased that this was his manner of showing that he cared about me and giving me hope about myself. He prescribed new glasses, shook hands with me, said I should return in two years, and wished me well.

I was once more very pleased. I had passed another milestone and kept my sense of being exactly myself. I could see now that part of my fear was based on my own conviction that I had changed because of the cancer, that I was no longer a person free of the terrible plague, that I was one of the lepers of the 20th century.

Dr. Stonewell gave me another indirect sign of his caring. My insurance covers routine checkups only in part. Dr. Stonewell had charged me the full fee in the past. The secretary said to me that he had indicated that I should be given a fifty percent courtesy discount. Amazed at the manner in which he gave me an indication of sympathy with my predicament, I gave her a check. His was the first indirect sign of caring. From now on many people, upon hearing of my cancer, would respond with indirect signs of caring: a friend sent me a delicate pendant; another took me to see a play; a third one gave me a subscription to a magazine; a fourth one gave me a plant; a fifth gave me a funny shopping bag for my errands. I learned the depth of feeling that could be condensed in a myriad of small gestures and gifts. In an act of humble acceptance of human love and human pain, I began to wear my gifts with the pride of a soldier wearing decorations for actions in the battlefield. I collected other gifts as the sportswoman collects trophies for her athletic feats. I had a shelf in the den full of treasures, from crystal vases that came with a rosebud to paper weights made by hand by an artist in a foreign land. They stood there like small monuments to the varieties of the experience of human compassion, small voices of human companionship for the days to come in the journey of my life.

October 4

My moods were like a see-saw. One day I felt enthusiastic and found myself dreaming about my future. I though of myself 85 years old, having a lovely time, like Georgia O'Keeffe, exploring with an imaginary excursion group the majestic beauty of New Mexico. I seemed in my old age to be perfectly well and certainly not short of stamina. The next day I was looking, just in passing, at the mirror on the bathroom door when I woke up a few minutes later from a brief daydream in which I had seen my dead, sunken, ravaged face, fixed by death, encased in a coffin. I was, like Tom Sawyer, attending my own wake. I was in the coffin, looking and dressed exactly as I did at the moment I was fantasizing it.

Caught between fantasies of enjoyable longevity and visions of imminent death was an even more frightening and repeated image of a woman wasting away in a dark nursing home, alone, immensely sad, very weak, her eyes bulging with uncertainty and vigilant fear.

I had no power over these daydreams. They came upon me like small strips of film, flashing their sunny or gloomy colors in front of my mind's eye and gripping my feelings with the force of their vivid images.

I learned from them that I wanted to hope as much as I was afraid of hoping, that I was trying to anticipate, to prepare myself to endure the horrors to come. I also discovered that these insistent daydreams kept me from getting back into things, from committing my heart to my real life, the one I had at hand today.

I wavered between impotence and compassion for myself. The impatient me kept saying, "Come on. You *had* cancer. Stop behaving as though you are half a corpse. Get on with your life." The compassionate me talked like a mother to a little girl, "Do not be so scared. You are well now. Maybe you will never be ill with cancer again. It is all right to see coffins and a dying you. That is your fear. You are *not* dying now or in the immediate future. Come! Let's go back to your homework."

Some days I succeeded in listening to the compassionate me, and, distracted by the comfort of feeling attended to by my inner voices, I would immerse myself in work, my chores, my dialogues with friends, and come out of all this full of joy, sensing that I was there where the action was. Other days, however, I had to muster all the will power I had at hand to force myself to do what I had to do while feeling that it was all an act of self-deception, letting myself believe that it made no difference that I go on with my life, that one fateful morning I would feel a sharp pain in my back and that would be the beginning of my destruction by metastatic cancer. "Give up; give up," a sordid, muted voice said mockingly. "Don't fool yourself." In those days I had to behave as Amundsen had in his march toward the South Pole, pushing on, one foot after the other, on the frozen and treacherous ground, aiming at my goal for the moment or the day, regardless of hopelessness, fatigue, fear. I had no South Pole to conquer, but I had to keep my little planet, my life territory, under control.

While my heart was oscillating in this wild manner, my body seemed to be doing its mending with simple faithfulness. Each day it gave me a new gift of energy, that indefinable bodily feeling that one has what it takes to go around minding one's own business. One afternoon I had so many errands to run after my work in the office that I decided to leave immediately after the last patient had gone. I had a list in my hand and dashed from one thing to the next. Suddenly, while I was in the middle of a store trying to buy some pantyhose, I realized with amazement that for the first time since the beginning of chemotherapy I had not had a nap in the middle of the afternoon. To crown with joy the surprise of my discovery, I realized that I was not feeling tired even though it was almost suppertime.

That was another milestone in my march toward recovery. I felt elated because my body was showing, without the demand of my will, that it was getting ready for all I wanted it to do. I recalled the words of Monique, who had said repeatedly that I would not begin to feel well until two to two and a half months after the last dose of chemotherapy. It was now 10 weeks since my last treatment. The confirmation of her prediction recalled other predictions that Dr. Nagle had made. I could expect to be free of metastasis for five years, perhaps for ten, maybe forever. The resurrection of my body seemed to give credibility to the resurrection of the rest of me. My gloom went down a few notches.

From that moment on, my body's messages were all good news. Sensations, feelings I had forgotten I could experience, presented themselves with the freshness of dew. I began to sleep deeply, restfully, with abandonment. My skin seemed to be more alert, to envelop me in a relaxed lining of warm comfort. My head cleared up from an indefinable cloud that I seemed to have carried mostly in my frontal or parietal lobes. I seemed to have a better grasp of everything. The feeling could be compared to the clear air of a spring morning when objects and shapes acquire a definition of form, a radiant luminosity. Food tasted better with a depth of flavor that the chemotherapy had obliterated. I was no longer nauseated, that persistent feeling of disgust for some unnamed content of the stomach. My appetite decreased.

I no longer had to get up at three in the morning to eat. I did not have to pop antacid tablets all day long to control gastric acidity, even though I needed one every so often if I skipped a scheduled meal. The shortness of breath while walking became less and less everyday. I still had 14 extra pounds that I had gained as the combined result of lack of exercise and excessive eating. The new message of my body, the report that it had the stamina to take me around, was the unexpected signal I was waiting for to try to lose those pounds I hated so much. I had always been slim, and I could not recognize myself as a plump person. Now I had the green light to diet and exercise to bring my faithful, good servant body to a more shapely look. The experience, the thoughts, the surprise, the joy of this first day without a nap, made it like another of those days at the beginning of creation when God saw that He had brought forth good things.

October 11

The time had come to return to the activities I had left behind. I began attending some professional meetings, social gatherings, and cultural activities. On each occasion, I found myself anxious, preoccupied with signals that I might unknowingly give out that would inform people that I had cancer. I was like a criminal who fears that her own actions will give her away. I found myself vigilant, unspontaneous, checking my reactions, and watching colleagues and acquaintances watching me in a double game of mutual espionage. Each time the remarks of other people indicated that they knew nothing, I experienced great relief. When people told me after attentively looking at my face that I looked very well, I found myself in a cloud of confusing feelings: pleasure that I had not betrayed the secrets of my recent illness and guilt that I was fooling them, cheating in the business of honest human commerce. I had frequent daydreams about their "catching" me. I saw "them" learning in some future time that I was dying of metastatic cancer or hospitalized for it, and "they" shook their heads, saying in disbelief, "She concealed it so well. It's unbelievable that she did not say anything when I asked her how she was." A voice coming from remote corners of an imaginary courthouse said solemnly, "She is found guilty of betrayal." Hearing the verdict, I felt ashamed of my duplicity, of my lack of candor with many people who cared about me.

Soon after, the voice of reason spoke softly but firmly, "You have the right to privacy. You can go freely about your business with these people if they don't know about your illness, if cancer is not in between you and them."

Finally, the natural flow of everyday life took over my worries and concerns and blended them with the task at hand until I was back to myself, fully doing what I was doing. When the chattering of a dinner party had me truly involved in a conversation or a scientific discussion found me eagerly defending my point of view, I realized that I had crossed the moat around my castle and joined my fellow human beings.

I had other concerns when I attended a function and had to relate to some people who knew in detail about my cancer and others who did not. I was afraid that a mild and caring gesture that they could not help making would betray that "something" was the matter with me. One night I got furious with the wife of a colleague who, in the midst of a crowded party, began asking me direct questions about my illness. I could barely contain my anger. I managed, however, to say calmly, "Let's not talk about that here. Let's talk about it privately." Others gave me more reasons to worry. I found myself getting smarter by the minute in handling these minor risk situations. One day a colleague said to the secretary of the department where I teach part time, "Dr. Meldin is not feeling well." It was a happy coincidence that I *did* have a cold and thus was able to use elegant sophistry in talking later to the secretary. I laughed and said that Dr. Zelyp was exaggerating a little and that "a cold will not kill me if I do a little extra work" but that I was delighted that somebody else was doing it.

On another occasion, a secretary who had to be informed and who was capable of handling a secret gave out an unwitting sign. I went to a lecture that was very important for the department. She came to greet me and said with her most compassionate expression, "I am so glad you could make it." I knew she was speaking from the depth of her feeling and that there was no malice in her, no ill intent to make my predicament public. I found myself responding creatively, once more on the edge of truth, "I am glad too. I thought I could never make it. Happily they fixed my *car* just at the last minute," I said winking. She understood and said immediately, "I know. Car troubles can be such a nuisance." We both knew that "I know" meant she knew that she should not have been so expansive at seeing *me* fixed and knowing what we both knew. We smiled sympathetically at each other. Shakespeare was certainly more than right in saying that life is a play and that we ordinary human beings can be very good actors and actresses.

True pain came with meeting old friends who had neglected me completely, withdrawing in horror (and sorrow?) upon learning of my cancer. My friend Harold, a colleague and friend of many years, 20 at least, had dashed to the hospital two days after the mastectomy, as soon as he learned what had happened. He could barely talk and left, mumbling something, after a couple of minutes. Neither he nor his wife called again. In the past we had shared trips abroad full of adventure and fun. We had shared our careers, the successes, the worries and failures. We had talked about their children growing and about my not having them. We had chatted about the manifold vicissitudes of life—political, social, and domestic. We had shared values and concerns. We had done all that with joy and with conviction. Now, in the dark hour of my cancer, they had left me alone to walk by myself down the dark corridor of chemotherapy and plastic surgery.

Harold and Nina, his wife, became a dull and constant pain for me, a pain that became acute the day I met Harold at a lecture given by a mutual friend who had extended his affection to me during the long months of treatment. My good feelings for Manfred and my interest in his lecture were clouded by the fear of having to meet Harold face to face. I did not want to see him. I was full of resentment because I felt rejected, disregarded, discarded, as though I had been used as a friend when I was well and capable of laughter and fun and then disposed of as a broken toy.

I dreaded the moment when I had to greet him. I feared I would say something truly awful. I tried my best to rehearse the sentences that would modulate my resentment at the moment we met.

He came over as though nothing had happened. He smiled broadly and shook my hand vigorously. I did not want to embarrass him or myself in front of many colleagues and friends. I held his hand, pulled him near, and said softly, "Harold, we have to talk." At that moment someone came to greet us·both and nothing else could be said. Harold turned around and left before I had time to make any further contact with him. I waited 48 hours, hoping he would call me, take the initiative to have some dialogue. He did not, nor did his wife. The contrast with the past was shocking. He had been in the habit, before

I became a cancer case, of calling me with great excitement about some advance in his work, some special event in the family, or something that he knew I was doing.

My anguish increased by the hour. Alongside the hurt and the resentment was the painful feeling that I was losing a friend of many years, a friend who was my colleague and whom I had to see and deal with all the time. I reflected about the best course to take. Finally, it occurred to me that the best I could do was to leave a message on his office answering machine during the weekend. I knew that he checked the tape once a day. If I told him what was the matter, it would give him time to reflect and decide what to do.

Late at night on Friday, knowing that he would not be in the office, I called and left my message, "Harold, this is a continuation of what I said on Wednesday night. We have to talk. We cannot behave as though nothing has happened. I have too many feelings about not seeing you during all this time. Please do call." Saturday went by with no calls at all. I was as afraid that he would call as I was that he wouldn't. I did not know what to do with him or with myself. I went to sleep heavy hearted.

That night I had a nightmare. I was getting undressed when I saw that I had a hole in the nipple of my good breast. A white, puslike material oozed out of it. I looked closer and found that I had an open wound under the nipple. More whitish material came out of it. Suddenly the breast burst open, and yellowish liquid came out of the wound with the gurgling sound of a bottle that is being emptied. I looked in horror and witnessed the breast being deflated like a broken balloon. I could see the skin of the breast wrinkling and folding over the chest wall. I ran to the phone to call the plastic surgeon, who asked me to go to the hospital at once.

I found myself in a city I had known as a young woman. I had no car. I took a bus and got off at a stop in a residential neighborhood. I took many wandering streets, walking with difficulty up a narrow street on a hill. The hospital was strange. It looked like a prison I had seen in a T.V. show or perhaps like a hospital in a Swedish movie. The patients were all tall and pale, all women. The nurses were stern. I was frightened. I wandered through corridors and finally found a room for myself. It was the wrong room. The nurse came, took me to see the common bathroom — like that in a boarding school — and finally took me to my room. I was frightened. I wanted to see my doctor at once.

There were no doctors at hand. The nurse told me to get into bed. I could hear other patients moaning. I noticed that all of them wore white caps and long white gowns. The nurse asked me to put on a gown and a cap. She smiled. I couldn't. I felt too frightened to do anything but obey orders. The dream became confused at this point. When I woke up I was lost, wandering in the hospital neighborhood trying to get back to the hospital. Apparently I had left and couldn't find my way back. My first thought at the moment of awaking was, "I have not talked to my doctor."

October 18

My wish to talk to Harold had another source too, besides the need to find resolution for a painful situation. The source was another wish that was growing stronger by the day. It was a wish for closure, for completing a chapter, for turning a leaf in the book of my life. I wanted to go on with whatever was at hand. I became impatient and irritable when I had to keep repeating that I was well and that I was now back to most of my activities. I did not want to focus all conversation about me on my physical health. I wanted the rest of me to take its share. I wanted to attend to my ideas, to the work I was doing, to plans and dreams I was beginning to have again. I was also frightened of dreaming, of thinking that I had a future and that I could plan things like everybody else. In my fear, I needed to talk with my friends as ordinary people do about some real or foolish dream or desire. It does not really matter if one can fulfill it or not. The dream itself is a delightful pleasure. Those who are healthy, not cancer patients, can indulge in the silliest of fantasies. They can talk about going to Moscow and crossing Russia by train, and friends will join them in their foolishness as though everyone were ready to pack up and go. But if I said I wanted to go to Orlando, Florida, I could see the eyes turning to check the color of my cheeks and question whether I should go or not. Nobody says anything, but the air can get heavy with unspoken thoughts and feelings, including my own.

No, I did not want to go on this way, like an invalid, an object of concern and worry. I wanted to close, as much as it could be closed, the chapter of my cancer. I had completed the "job." Whatever had to be removed had been removed. I had taken into my system all the chemotherapy I was told to take. I had had my anatomy remodeled as best as a human shape can be. I had done it all. "Now," I said, "it is done." It was time to go on, with fear, with trepidation, knowing that cancer could return any minute. I was not willing to spend my life waiting. I did not want to be like one of those New England widows of sea captains lost at sea, walking her widow's walk, day and night, scanning the horizon for the return of her husband.

No. I wanted to be reengaged with life, with laughter, with work, with silliness, with absurd fantasies, with commitments. I did not want the cancer to be the axis my life moved around. I wanted to be that axis, I, the person who had the cancer.

My impatience grew by the minute. I began telling my friends, sometimes to my surprise, that I was well now and that unless I get metastasis I would have no news to report. I was shocked at my way of talking but pleased too. The pleasure seemed to be the complex result of my having found a way of saying that they should stop asking me about my health. It was also the growing conviction that I was going to have time for myself, at least for a while. I noticed that I had some adolescent feelings of entering a new world, of dealing with new things I did not yet know, except that they were new. In fact, there was nothing new I could think about that was coming my way. I had to acknowledge to myself that the novelty was in the feeling itself, in realizing—I was shocked at my own thought—that I *had not died of cancer*.

My thoughts returned to Gospel imagery and the side of the Gospels nobody says anything about. The miraculously resurrected son of the widow of Naim came to mind. What did he feel? What did he think? How did he perceive the world after having died in his youth? How did he perceive his own life after death? How did he feel about not being dead? What was the color, the smell, the flavor of life for him? Did he feel the same wish, after his extraordinary return to life, to go back to the ordinary routine of everyday? Did he, like me, want to eat simple meals without being looked at? Did he wish to be like everybody else and not a resurrected one? What do we, the not-yet-dead or the dead-come-back, want? I imagined him saying sadly, "I want to be the young man I used to be before I died. I want to grow and marry and have children. I am glad the Lord performed a miracle for me, but I do not want to be the resurrected one anymore."

I applauded his little speech with enthusiasm. I noticed I was the only one applauding while the others looked on with incredulous eyes.

"He is right," I said addressing them. "I know he is right. I did not die, but I had cancer, which is quite deadly as you know." The unusual crowd of first century Jews and my friends nodded sadly, respectfully. "Neither he, with his resurrected body, nor I, with my body free of cancer for today, wants you all to look at us with those big, compassionate, amazed eyes. He and I want you to look at us as you look at everybody else. Yes, that is what we want." The young man echoed vehemently, "Yes, that is what we want. After all," he said, sadly confronting them, "I am alive today exactly the same way *you* are alive." A muted, contained exclamation passed over the crowd like the wind over the fields of wheat, ruffling minds and bodies. "I want you," I said valiantly, "to accept that for today our lives—yours and those of this young man and mine—are truly alike. We are not different from you. Do not segregate us, neither in your acts nor in your minds."

The crowd consented with a deep, pained, grunting noise, as though they were being asked to erase differences that jumped to the eye, like black and white, as though it were right not to discriminate between colors or between life and death.

The young man and I looked at each other and after a moment of hesitation, embraced one another in an affectionate gesture of solidarity.

The crowd gasped and then unexpectedly broke into laughter. Tears came to my eyes. The young man wiped his. I said shyly but firmly, "Thank you. Thank you."

Suddenly I felt that something real and essential had happened, some critical instant of transformation for all of us involved.

November 1

Now that I had regained my life, I had to keep it. Friends of every kind came up with the latest in cancer prevention, from dieting to the use of mental imagery. I collected a small library of books, pamphlets, newspapers, clippings, and American Cancer Society newsletters. The society had always sent me, as a licensed physician in practice, all its reports. I used to read them "for the benefit of those who have cancer," so as to be well informed about such a critical subject. Now the ink of their pages was running *for me.*

From every corner of the world the messages came like strident trumpets announcing significant events: I had a way of fighting or preventing cancer. *I* could do something. I *should* do something. "Now," I said to myself, "you have to follow the ten commandments of cancer-free heaven." I tried to list them following the old-fashioned Ten Commandments.

The first commandment, "I am the Lord your God; you shall have no other gods" was an easy one. I liked it, and I did not dare to change it. I was willing to put myself in the hands of the Lord. It was rather simple to let God do His loving job.

The trouble came with the second commandment. It was now my turn to do or not to do. "You shall not take the name of the Lord your God in vain." I decided to work out my cancer laws in a loose way, as best I could. I knew that God would not be offended by my taking the liberty of tampering with the Law to make an ad hoc set of commandments for my cancer pilgrimage. My God is not jealous but patient and compassionate with those who are frightened and at their wits' end. After all, Jesus himself was at his wit's end just before he died. My table of the law was a white piece of paper waiting for my new laws. After a long pause, it came to me ready made: *Do not use the word "cancer" in vain; it is neither so terrible nor so good a name.*

Now that I had written my own second cancer commandment, the others followed with the same ease I used to recite God's commandments in one breath in Sunday School.

"Remember the Sabbath Day. Six days you shall labor, but the seventh day is a Sabbath to the Lord." This one was the best. I enjoyed writing it. *Take time for your rest, not only on the sabbath but whenever you need it, be it with a friend or by yourself. Work, but do not let work dominate your life. Remember that you are alive and life deserves to be enjoyed for what it is, in contemplation and action.*

(I was pleased to notice how well I was moving along.)

The fourth commandment became: *Honor your father and mother and your siblings by working out your grudges against them. Resentment, anger, and depression will ruin your immune system and kill you.* The fourth commandment also brought good old Freudian conflict to the fore. "*Honor your father and your mother that your days may be long.*" The voices of the psychiatric and cancer literature sounded at this moment like thunder saying with solemn gravity: *Make peace with people around you. Resolve your grudges, your resentments, your anger, or otherwise your life will be short. Your immune system will know you haven't done it and your life will be shortened.* I felt like a minuscule sinner asked to repent of tremendous and horrifying crimes. It was a situation of "either/or," do or die. I felt stubborn, angry. I did not want to have to honor and forgive to save my life. I noticed I was even challenging the Lord for saying "that your days may be long." I did not want to have to exchange the currency of honor and forgiveness as a token for life. I felt the indignation of Moses when his people let him down, and from this rebellious mood came the fourth commandment. *Honor all living creatures, your fellow humans and yourself, because there is a mystery in it all that you can't possibly grasp. Honor them all with simple reverence.* I was surprised and a bit alarmed. I feared my critics. This was not sounding much like cancer commandments according to the books. I silently promised to do my best to turn them into real cancer commandments.

The fifth gave me an easy break to keep my promise. "You shall not kill." I wrote at once, *Do not kill yourself with the wrong food. Eat well. Exercise. Have your checkups. Be alert, and love yourself. Do not be a goody-goody, because it could do you harm. Speak your mind. Burp your grudges as soon as you get them.*

The sixth said, "Do not commit adultery." I laughed. In my situation adultery was rather a difficult task. The magazine article writers and the cancer saviors did not like my laughter, so I hurried to write the commandment that had come to me. I had to use a bit of slang. *Do not fornicate against yourself; do not f_____ yourself with morbid thoughts. Have wonderful fantasies about yourself, your world. Make love to yourself.* I tried to lower my face. I was afraid that the saviors could see the little twinkle at the corner of my eye. To cover up, I hurried to the seventh commandment.

"You shall not steal." I felt virtuous cancerwise, writing my own version. *Do not steal good times, good things, good laughter from yourself. Do what is best for you.* I must say I like it very much that everybody agreed that I should pamper myself. I decided I was going to be firm with any pangs of guilt when impatient voices from the past accused me of selfishness. I think this is a great commandment.

The eighth commandment came along. "You shall not bear false witness against your neighbor." This one reminded me at once of the poor woman who had come at 10:00 P.M. with her fake rose and her acrylic breast just before my discharge from the hospital after the mastectomy. My commandment came out of me with righteous determination. *Talk the plain truth about cancer with your neighbor. Do not sugar coat it. Do not falsify either its reality or its gravity. Do not mislead your neighbor.* At that moment I felt that even when my professional situation required great discretion, I would make myself available to talk to people with cancer whom I would meet through private channels. I would not bear false witness against my fellow cancer friends and acquaintances.

The ninth command rolled along. "You shall not covet your neighbor's house or anything that is your neighbor's." This was a hard one. I did covet my neighbor's health, my women neighbors' breasts, my fellow human beings' unthreatened lives. I could not lie here. I could not write a false commandment, so I wrote what I could do. *I shall ask every day of my life to accept humbly what I still have and to be patient with myself when I find myself wanting what my neighbor has.*

The tenth commandment made me laugh again "You shall not covet your neighbor's wife." I decided I could stay with only nine commandments because in my heart of hearts I knew that whenever I saw my neighbor's very nice husband, I would without question covet him. I also knew that my wish for a nice husband would not go beyond the bittersweet reality of my being alone. So it was that I gave myself permission to have wishful fantasies without adultery. The cancer prevention people frowned a little at this permission to have fantasies that were not directly aimed at killing metastatic cells or bringing me to the highest peak of health. They seemed to agree that I was not a good client. I was too rebellious, too independent minded. After looking at each other, they let me keep my tenth commandment as it was. They seemed to believe that there was nothing they could do to improve my stubbornness, to make me more serious in handling anticancer wishes and to encourage me to give up silly fantasies about imaginary husbands.

The commandments, once I wrote them down, appeared to me as a very mixed law to live by.

I could say in all honesty that I had practiced several of them without knowing that they were supposed to protect me from cancer. For ten years I had eaten in such a way – vegetable, fruit, cereals, grains, white meat, skim milk, calcium (for osteoporosis), no junk food or drinks – that I could win a dietetic society's first prize. When my body fat was checked several years ago as a part of a research project, I came out a winner. The doctor and the research nurse said with shining eyes that I had, for a woman of my age (44) the lowest fat content in the curve, that I was made out of good, solid muscle. I had never smoked. I had never drunk more than a glass of wine now and then. I had always exercised. I had – I must confess humbly – been a goody-goody in the sense that I liked to do things well and, more frequently than not, I preferred to be kind to others. I do not think, however, that that prevented me from speaking my mind. So, on weighing the factors on the scale of good-goody/speak up, I think I came out even. I shall not go on describing how I have obeyed most of the anticancer commandments, including having every medical checkup I was supposed to have.

According to these commandments I was *not supposed* to have had cancer, that is, if one regards them as a superstition, a talisman to exorcise evil cells. Nevertheless I did have cancer. The voices of those who gave the commandments rose like a roaring sea wave, "True, true, but you detected it early. Your prognosis is good. You caught it in time. Do not complain. Keep on obeying the commandments."

"Yes," I said out of superstitious and rational fear and a little bit out of conviction. "Yes, you know I did obey them, and I will continue to do so."

Then male and female voices with slightly theatrical pitches twice asked rhetorically, "What about imagery? What about imagery?"

I lowered my head in shame. They had caught me. I was not using imagery. It was not out of ignorance. I had in my head and on the shelves of my bedroom book stand every book and article that had been published. They had failed to convince me. I had tried to follow some of their suggestions, and I was not able to make them compatible with me, the whole person I am.

During chemotherapy I was supposed to imagine the work of the drugs as bullets or something else. It did not make sense to me. To me – the me I am – I was involved in a tragic drama of life and death, one of the many profound tragedies of life in which we use heroic measures: killing our own cells with chemotherapy to preserve our life. I am a serene realist. That was the reality, and I was willing to see it and live it in its depth of drama, pain, conflict and hope. Chemotherapy was not an electronic game of bullets hitting targets. It was the unavoidable tragedy and pain of being human and mortal that I had to face as any other human being had had to do since the beginning of time. I am not able to transform a threat of death into playful imagery. I needed to face *me* caught in the potential grip of a frightening death. I needed to accept that, like the heroes of all times, I had to take my journey with trepidation and courage, knowing all along that to save myself I had to go through an ordeal of horror and pain and even to risk losing life itself.

My listeners seemed to have heard my thoughts. They now spoke softly but firmly.

"You are now free of cancer. Won't you try imagery, meditation, biofeedback, and perhaps (they seemed to have heard me saying that I did obey their commandments before I found my cancer) remain free of cancer?"

This time I could see they had a point. They were not telling me to use electronic game imagery to kill murderous cells. They were telling me to reflect on life, to find life-sustaining, meaningful measures to support me, *me*, body, mind, and soul in my way of being. I had to agree with them. I tried to be humble. "I'll try the best I can," I said, honestly measuring my words. I had to agree with them that it was essential for me to protect my life from unnecessary stress and to create for myself an optimal situation to enhance my improved health and diminish any unnecessary risk.

I knew enough about the workings of the immune system to see that there could be a relation between stress and the immune system's inability to free the body from abnormal cells or invasive germs. It made eminent sense that I had to help my body and my immune system to help me.

The point was clear. The decision was now about the means to achieve it. My friends returned with new books and articles, names of consultants, stories of modern scientific miracles, and other witnesses, whose words sounded remarkably close to Christian Scientist or Baptist healings without belief in a healing God.

A businessman went from his deathbed to a full recovery. A housewife emerged from postcancerous chronic depression to a life of great satisfaction and relaxation. Numerous more sober witnesses spoke about their imaging, meditation, or biofeedback. Meditation seemed to be a favorite of many. Others were "high" on imaging. A few suggested biofeedback. I pointed out that I had no specific symptoms to deal with that called for biofeedback. At this point, if one excluded a little bit of postchemotherapy fatigue, I seemed and was the portrait of health, a slightly plump health but health anyway. The only use of biofeedback would be to relax. "So," I asked myself, "do I need to relax? Am I not relaxed? Do I have to train myself in relaxation to exorcise metastasis?" I did not know the answer to this question. I had to give myself time to provide it.

November 8

To be fair to my friends and all the people who suggested transcendental meditation and relaxation, I read again Dr. Herbert Benson's *The Relaxation Response.* I came out of the reading pleased with his conclusions. The one that pleased me the most read, "changes consistent with the elicitation of relaxation response have been noted during the *imagined* [my emphasis] emotional experiences of reverence, love and grief" (p. 73). The next conclusion that gave me pleasure insisted that "the subject's attitude toward the exercise, and this is absolutely essential, must not be intense and compulsive, but of a 'let it happen' nature called 'passive concentration' " (p. 72).

Dr. Benson has a whole chapter demonstrating that throughout history, men (he does not quote women and lost some points with me for it) of all ages, all convictions, all nations have discovered and practiced the relaxation response as part of their beliefs in their search for an encounter with a divine being or reality or inner peace.

Finally he concludes that

> the relaxation response is a universal human capacity, and even though it has been evoked in the religions of both East and West for most of recorded history, you don't have to engage in any rites or esoteric practices to bring it forth. The experience of the relaxation response has faded from our everyday life with the waning of religious practices and beliefs, but we can easily regain its benefits [p. 123].

Dr. Benson convinced me. He made eminent sense. Human beings do have an "inborn capacity" (p. 125) to enter a relaxation response, be it as a means to find spiritual integrity and a divine presence or simply to evoke some brain activity in the service of more earthly purposes.

From hindsight I recognized that I too had had many relaxation-response experiences, particularly when sitting alone, quietly, in the woods, near a stream, and passively letting the universe, in all its majesty and simple beauty, impress itself upon my being. I recalled how I used to love, and still love now, to sit on a stone at sunset or sunrise and let all my senses feel, without making any effort to perceive anything but concentrating on the simple act of being there, breathing rhythmically in synchrony with all that lives, "visible and invisible." Those are moments I always seek and "need." If I do not have them, I feel a great loss. "Alas!" I said to myself, "You have been having relaxation responses all your life without knowing it!" I was like the man who had spoken prose all his life unaware of his literary achievement.

Now that I had begun to like Dr. Benson's and his followers' suggestions, I was more than delighted that I was a "natural" for it. My self-contentment met the kind index finger of Dr. Benson and his coauthor, Miriam Z. Klipper, pointing at me as they said, "You know the experience. You know what it feels like. It won't do you lasting good if you experience it ten times in the summer. You *must* do it everyday if it is to make a difference in your life."

I felt like a child found out trying to skip doing the dishes or making her bed every day. "You are right," I said meekly, feeling torn between knowing that they were right and my fear that now I had to add another scheduled "thing" to the clock-run life I was already leading. My profession requires my being there exactly on the dot of the hour to meet my patients. I wanted to do it and get my relaxation response, and I did not want to do it. I wanted the great serenity that comes with the experience; I did not want the obligation of having to have it.

Once more Dr. Benson insisted that the regularity of doing it made the difference. He was joined by monks of every conviction, East and West, saying that disciplined faithfulness to the practice was indispensable.

"You are right," I said again, a bit more crestfallen this second time. I did not want to give in. I became argumentative. "How do you," I said with brave intensity, "sleep eight hours a day, see eight patients a day, read and answer your correspondence and telephone, pay your bills, attend to your house, see your friends, do the shopping, watch the news, read the newspapers, do your hair, wash, exercise, move your bowels, and attend to uninvited daily catastrophes, all of it in 24 hours, and still add two periods of 20 minutes a day to save your life with a beautiful relaxation response?" I got short winded with my own long sentence. I caught my breath and said defiantly, like a rascal who has life-saving evidence, "All that adds up to 35 hours a day!" Dr. Benson shook his head with compassionate despair. It was becoming clear that I was a very stubborn character, perhaps destined to kill myself with mismanaged stress. He said nothing. I felt embarrassed and responded to his thoughts, "I know. I know," I said, "But still. . . ." I did not complete the sentence.

I was now thinking about the first sentence that had impressed me. Even imagined experiences of reverence, love, and grief could bring about "changes consistent with the relaxation response" (p. 73). That had a chance for me. I am very resistant to bringing about changes in myself by acts, no matter how relevant, like the relaxation response, that are not part of the very core of life, the very essentials of the act of living. Reverence, love, and grief are, in my experience, at the very core of our God-given mortal and humanly bonded life. If they brought about the relaxation response, I was a natural for it. Reverence, in fact, is one of the things I would like to have more of. I had no choice but to have grief, facing, as I had to, the reality of having had a truly mortal cancer. Love is something that needs no time. As a matter of fact the best thing about those three is that they require no time set aside, and they encompass all the time we have to do what we have to do. Reverence is the simplest of them all. It only requires a great sense of wonder, respect, simplicity, and admiration in dealing with the marvels of all God and man made things, from little spiders with lacy webs to telephones carrying a tiny human voice in two seconds from Baghdad to New York.

Therefore I made a vow to practice, from awakening to falling asleep, the act of reverence that life deserves.

Then, remembering my Christian learning—and not without a prayer for help and grace—I made a vow to love all creatures great and small, *good and bad*, as my fellow travelers in the trip of life.

Finally, trembling like a leaf about to be blown off of the tree by a fall breeze, I vowed to grieve the loss of my life, whenever it might come. I vowed to accept death.

I felt that my vows were good, that they were at the essence of the two unavoidable acts I *had* to carry out: to live and to die.

I wanted, however, to be fair to Dr. Benson, who had taught me much with his book. I looked at him, his finger no longer pointing at me, and said, "Whenever I can, I will do the 20-minute technique you recommend on page 114. I will place a small chair in the little room in the attic where there is absolute peace and quiet and go there for the relaxation." I said it seriously. He smiled like a man used to rebellious souls who little by little come to understand that what he has to offer is good.

With this resolution, I discovered that I did not want the gimmicks of imagery. If reverence, love, and grief are truly genuine emotions, the imagery that comes with them must be more than enough to sustain a meaningful life, to prepare me for a meaningful death, be it death by cancer or by any other way, whenever the time came for me to surrender my life.

November 9

Yesterday I was talking about surrendering my life. Today I remember my friend Elizabeth, who would not give hers up before seeing again the lake of our youth. At the time of our last encounter she had given me a bottle of local liqueur she knew I like very much. After her death, whenever I felt a need for her, I went to the bar in the living room and served myself a very small measure of the liqueur. Thinking about my death brought tears to my eyes about her premature death. As I had done before, I went to the bar for my encounter with her, to renew our friendship through her gift. The bottle had the last measure for my small glass. It was almost two years to the day that Elizabeth had died. I drank very slowly, savoring the drink and her friendship. I recalled a short story, I do not know by whom, that I read a long time ago. The storyteller describes the final disappearance of the traces a man has left in life when a clerk in an obscure government office is crossing out names of deceased people and destroying the documents carrying their names. The clerk looks briefly at the man's folio, and, after crossing out the name with red ink in a log book, he throws the folio into the waste basket. The man's name, written in large print, can be read from the paper sticking out of the basket. The writer closes the story, saying, "That was the last time anyone saw his name."

I had the feeling I was burying Elizabeth again. I had not been able to attend her funeral. I felt that throwing out the bottle was like a little funeral, another and more final way of burying what she had touched with her living hands. I found myself crying, a few tears rolling down my cheeks. I kissed the bottle tenderly, as I would have kissed her face had I been able to go to her wake. "Bye, Elizabeth," I said, and, feeling the tenderness of Shakespeare, I added, "Bye, sweet Elizabeth, sweet friend and companion." I deposited the bottle carefully in the waste basket in the kitchen, sensing the finality of my act and of death. I turned around full of grief, knowing that I still had a few things left that Elizabeth had given me for us to continue our friendship.

November 15, morning

I did it. I went to my hairdresser. I tricked myself. I knew that if I walked by the shop on a Tuesday afternoon I probably would find him free, and we could do it all at once, without appointments and preambles. I was like a person who has committed a crime and fears that some little detail will give her away. I imagined, in spite of myself, numerous sessions where he caught me with my cancer. "What has happened to your hair?" he asked in my mind. "It is all damaged." Or he asked, "Have you been ill? Your hair is not normal. Are you eating well?" Daniel, the hairdresser, is a truly gentle and respectful man, but in this scenario he looked stern and impatient like the hairdresser who said to my mother when I was five, "This child has impossible hair. I don't know what to do with her."

As soon as I came out of my fantasies, I gave myself a few pep talks. "Don't be silly. Your hair is normal. It did *not* fall out. Nothing is different. He cannot notice anything. If he does, tell him you didn't realize there was anything wrong. Ask him what it is." I managed, while I was walking in the direction of his shop, to do other errands to calm myself for a while. Then I started all over again. I made myself aware that for this case of mine as for many others, the proof of the pudding was in the eating. I had to go and have it over with. This courageous resolution came to me when I was two buildings away from the beauty parlor. I marched now like a brave soldier to the front line, eyes high, legs firm, gathering my full voice for the first words.

Daniel was downstairs having a coffee break. The woman at the desk told him on the intercom that a customer wanted to see him. He came up in a few minutes and said he had not seen me in a long time.

I, feeling like Sarah Bernhardt, told my prepared lie casually, with proper intonation and naturalness, I said "I decided to change the hair style and let my hair grow."

"I see that it has grown quite a bit," Daniel said. "How long do you want it?"

"Well," I said, "that is why I came in to chat with you." He was now touching my hair, looking at its texture and length and trying to assess its condition. My heart was racing as though he could as well dispose of my life right there.

His verdict came. "It has grown a lot, but it is uneven. It would be best if you trim it a half-inch or an inch all around. It is much longer on the surface than underneath, and it does not look nice in the back. If I cut it all around, it would look very nice. Your hair is very natural, like a natural perm, and it would look nice. You should take advantage of it." His hand kept picking up different strands of hair and contemplating them carefully. "Yes," he concluded, "it would look very nice once trimmed."

I felt immensely relieved. Daniel and I had reestablished our relationship, and I had kept my secret with poised dignity.

Daniel began his work, skillfully trimming here and there, and then contemplated his work. After a while he said, "Your hair has more white now. Last year I told you not to dye it, but now it would be good to do it. You'll look younger." I confessed that two different friends had given me hair dye, the one they used, for me to try and that I was a coward because I had not got myself to do it. He suggested he could do it. The dye they use has peroxide, however, and I did not want that but something natural. He said that was fine, but that I should do it. Then, with a broad smile and expression of mischief, he said, "I have been doing it for ten years." I was amazed. He was a good 15 years younger than I and had dark, very curly hair. I looked at him, and truly one could not say that his hair betrayed any doctoring at all.

He was now proudly stretching out his dark hair to show how nice it looked and how the white hairs were completely disguised. "I'll try," I said. "I am going on a short vacation, and I will use the leisure time to learn how to do it." He said it was very easy; so had my friends. One of them, Carla, had given me a very comprehensive demonstration of how she covered the white strands of her long and abundant hair.

Nevertheless, I was a coward. I had always liked natural things, and no one in my family had ever needed to dye her hair. The women did not have gray hair until they were in their mid-seventies. My grand-father, my father, and now my mother were in their eighties before their hair became white. I think I was *offended* that according to those statistics I was graying prematurely. I was also afraid of a skin reaction. Frequently I have reacted to some ordinary cosmetics with very bad rashes. Finally, if I am truly honest, I was indignant that the stress of my cancer seemed to have contributed to the accelerated graying of my hair. It was like adding insult to injury.

Deep down I knew it was better for me to gather my wits and do it. "After all," I thought while Daniel was vigorously combing my hair, "it would make me look good and cover up–another cover up–the cancer chapter of my life." Daniel was now contemplating the end result of his work. He seemed pretty satisfied with my looks. "It looks very nice on you to have it at this length. After all, you have the right natural hair for it," he said. I felt proud of my "beauty" and immensely grateful that my reunion with Daniel had gone smoothly and that now I could come to see him without having to be crazy about it.

"You did a great job," I said, holding the mirror and contemplating the sculpting work Daniel had performed on my top. The hair encircled my head, curling around my ears, forehead and back. This was my real head and hair, free of terrible threats. I could be confident that my scalp would do its faithful job of making my hair grow, gray or not, but curly and silky.

"That's it," Daniel said. He gave me the slip for me to pay the cashier. "Come back when you want me to trim it again."

"Thank you, Daniel," I said, knowing he could not know the depth of joy and gratitude captured in those two words.

"Bye," he said and returned to his coffee break downstairs.

November 25, afternoon

On Thursday, Harold and I made peace with each other. He had called me on the Tuesday after the Friday I had left my message on his office telephone answering machine about needing to talk with him. We talked for a good while. He said he thought I wanted my privacy. I said that I had wanted his caring and that I had never before asked him to stay out of my life. He seemed to begin to understand something obscure about himself, and then, suddenly, without my help, he realized that we were talking about the difficulty on my part to keep him as a friend. He said sorrowfully, almost pleading, "We have been friends for almost 20 years. You are the person I always call when something good happens to me. You are always first on my list."

"Yes," I said, "I have always been first on your list when you needed me. This time I needed you, and you forgot about me. I needed your presence, your friendship, your visits, and you were nowhere to be found."

He was silent for a long time, and I had no more to say. Finally he said, "You are right. I don't know why I did not call or visit you. I said to myself that you wanted your privacy, but you never said that." His voice dropped a few decibels, "Do you still want me for a friend? I'll take you to lunch, and we'll talk."

"Harold," I said, "I cannot be your friend if I don't forgive you. I am too angry, too resentful, too disappointed with you. You have to convince me that I should forgive you."

"Give me a chance," he said quietly. "Let's find a time to have lunch together. I'll take you to the best place in town." We found that a Thursday, two weeks from the moment of the conversation, was a time when we both could go to lunch in the early afternoon. "I'll pick you up," he said.

I was as nervous as a girl on her first date. I was afraid that Harold would not give me a meaningful reason to forgive him, that he would gloss over the whole episode and ask me to make all the adjustments. I did not want him to humiliate himself, but I knew that his and my actions could acquire meaning only in their full integrity. He had to feel that forgiving him was a true continuation of friendship, not patching up or covering up resentful feelings. I needed him to give me proof that he understood he had failed me and that he regretted it.

I waited for the encounter with anxious preoccupation, not knowing how I would feel one way or the other.

Harold came at the exact minute we had agreed he would pick me up. We were both a bit stiff in greeting each other. We did not know whether to kiss or shake hands or what to say. We both said, "Hi!" with high pitched voices. We both used practical details to fill the air with words. "Let me put the alarm on," I said.

"Take your time. Do you need help to go to the car?" he asked.

"No, thank you. I am quite well now," I responded. He had a new

car. It was not a fancy model as before but a comfortable, standard car.
"Well," I said, "I see you are getting into America's everybody's car."

He laughed. "I've had it with all those foreign cars. They cost a
fortune to repair. You never find the right mechanic. My car always
broke down in the middle of nowhere, and nobody knew how to fix it.
I wanted to get a GM, a Chrysler, or a Ford. So I found this one. It is
inexpensive. It always works, and you find parts to repair it in every
garage even if you happen to be in the middle of the country."

"Yes," I said, "I know. I too am the happy owner of an old Ford. It
is laughable what it costs me to repair it." I touched the upholstery and
the front panel and looked at details of the car as a connoisseur. "It is
pretty nice," I said with genuine praise. "Comfortable. It has everything. What else do you need?"

He laughed, "Nothing. I am happy as a pig with it."

I laughed too. "Well," I said, picking up on his first indication of
relaxation, "I am as happy as Miss Piggy with mine. I am sticking to my
Ford like the most patriotic American trying to beat the Japanese car
industry." He laughed again. I felt we were carefully building a climate
for dialogue, bits of chit-chat to pave the way for the mending we had
to do.

Harold parked the car and took the lead. We found a good table
where we could talk freely without being overheard. We ordered and
chatted more about food and restaurants. I could feel the sadness
growing within me. Was Harold going to keep the conversation at this
level? Was he once more going to avoid dealing with me? Would I lose
him as a friend? I was close to tears. I kept munching bits of bread to
contain myself. I did not want to have to confront him again. I could
not force him to assume responsibility for our friendship. I began to
eat quietly, my nose in the dish, not knowing what to say.

Suddenly Harold leaned forward and said, "Madeleine , I have to
tell you what I learned about myself. I have done a lot of thinking.
Why did I treat you the way I did? Why did I avoid you? I could not
understand it myself. I never behaved this way. I have always been a
caring person. You know it."

"Yes," I said, "I know that."

"I have always been there when you needed me."

"Yes, you have."

"Then, why did I behave this way? I could not recognize myself.

Why? Why? Finally the other day I made the connection. It was the voice, your voice when you told me. Your voice was so full of sadness, so fatigued when you told me and when you talked to me at the hospital. What I discovered is that your voice sounded like my aunt Mary's voice when she got very ill before she died. I adored her. She was my favorite, like you. There is something in common between you and her. I was a teenager when she got sick. She lived in an apartment next door to ours. I used to visit her every afternoon when she was well. We talked and talked. She was so interesting. When she got sick, she changed. She was always fatigued, and her voice was low and sad. I stopped going. I couldn't get myself to go. My mother would try to help me to go and visit her. I would go, but it was too painful for me to stay. It is the only time in my life I avoided the pain of another person until I did it again with you. I have always been known for being the first one to be there when somebody needed me. I did not think I could do it again, but I did."

He paused. There was a long silence between us.

Finally I asked, "In what ways do I remind you of her?"

"I thought about that. I could talk with her in a way I couldn't talk with my parents. You are the same. I can talk with you. She listened. You do too. You are also alone, like her. She had no family of her own. She was always glad to see me. She had many stories, and I loved to hear them. When she got ill, it was a terrible loss for me. We couldn't talk anymore. I think I was afraid that the same would happen with you, that I would lose you. I know that in spite of all of this I should not have behaved the way I did with you. I am telling you this for you to understand how it happened that I did not behave like your friend. I have learned a lesson about myself. I have to watch myself from now on. Now I know I am capable of abandoning my friends."

Another long, intense silence gave weight to what Harold had said.

I was a bundle of confused feelings. I wanted to forgive him. I was afraid of forgiving him, afraid of a new betrayal. I was moved by his honesty and the soul-searching he had gone through. I was still angry and resentful. I was afraid of losing him as a friend and fearful of keeping him as a friend.

I made a great effort and asked him, "Did you think you were abandoning me, or you never thought of me?" He got upset.

"No. No. I thought about you all the time. Nina kept on asking me about you and saying that we should call you. I said that you wanted your privacy. That is what I found out about myself, that I made that up because I could not deal with you. I could not forget your voice when I visited you at the hospital. I was so upset. I just didn't know how to bring myself to talk with you. It was like with my aunt. I abandoned her too. It was my mother who made me go. I did not know what to do with myself when she was ill. I was not aware of what I was doing as I was not aware of my neglecting you. If you had not called me, asking me to explain myself, I would not have thought I did anything wrong, but I did. I was horrified when I realized how I had treated you. Now I have made a point. I have to watch myself. I could do this again."

"Then," I said, full of sorrow, "I could not forgive you."

"I hope," he said hurriedly, as though he wanted to capitalize on the momentum of my words, "I hope you forgive me this time."

"I want to forgive you," I said slowly, sadly, "but it is hard. It is hard to let the anger and the resentment go. I felt so neglected by you and Nina, as though you didn't care whether I lived or died."

He leaned a bit more towards me. "That is not true. No, that is not true. I thought about you all the time."

"But I didn't know it," I said impatiently. "How could I know you were concerned?"

"You couldn't. I have no excuse. I just told you what I found within me, the only explanation I can find for my behavior."

We both looked at our food and ate quietly. After a while he said, "I hope you'll give me another chance to prove that I care about you."

All of me did not want to forgive him. I wanted him to have his share of suffering, his own anguish for having failed a good friend. I wanted him to feel remorse and guilt, but I wanted to be a good friend too. It was now my turn to force myself to do what I knew I should do. My voice would not come out fully when I said the words, "I'll give you another chance."

He smiled sadly, stretched out his hand, and begged, "Forgive me." We shook hands.

"This is my official act of forgiveness," I said, and then with a cracking voice, "Please, Harold, do not let me down."

"I won't," he promised.

That was the moment when I found peace again with my friend Harold and myself. An enormous weight had been lifted from my shoulders. "Perhaps," I thought, "this very painful hour can deepen our friendship."

He took me home, and we kissed good-bye.

December 6

The anniversary of the day I found my breast lump had arrived quietly, unmarked, enmeshed in the business of everyday life.

I felt afraid of showering, superstitiously fearing that the gods had marked my other breast with cancer to create a sacred secret symmetry.

They had not. A sad mood settled on me and around me. I felt as though invisible beings, heralds of decay and death, fluttered around, their black wings vaulting around my body in silent formation. Muted cries and whispers came from the netherworld, carrying the lamentations of those transported to the secret chambers of death by cancerous disintegration. I felt like a damned soul, a marked body, a prisoner of the angel of death.

I could not shake the feeling of the fantasies. I went through the day without touching the ground, floating in the surrealistic space of those scheduled for death. My body felt unreal, strange, unrecognizable. It seemed strange that I was alive. It seemed strange that I was going from one task to another, working, talking to my patients, going to the bathroom, looking at my face in the mirror. I saw *the other one* looking at me from the mirror. She looked well, a bit round, a bit sad, and alive. Her cheeks were pink, her lips full, her eyes shiny, even in their sadness, her smooth forehead like a page ready for the new writings of life. She did not look like me, the terrified captive of a death squad. She looked like a middle-aged woman, poised, in good health, friendly, welcoming, comfortably installed in the office of life.

"Hey, you," I said to the woman in the mirror. "Are you me? What are you thinking? Talk, spirit, talk." I commanded now, "Talk!" and I waited.

She looked at me. Her face had become serious, almost contemplative. Her lips moved at their corners, slowly upwards. Her nostrils dilated with new air. Her eyes opened in tender wonderment. She tilted her head to the left just a little and then she said smilingly, "Do not be so frightened. You are well now. I do not see messengers of death around you. Let life take its course. Enjoy the life you have today. Let death come in its own time. Laugh with the joy of being alive, of having a warm body, touching hands, seeing eyes." She looked me in the eyes mischievously as though she knew that I needed her little speech to come back to my senses. We both laughed in unison.

The day continued with me in a mellow, sad mood. Every hour or so I would, in spite of my best efforts, recall the moment when my left hand found the fateful mass. The moment was imprinted on my mind with exquisite fidelity. I could remember every detail of that split second. I could recall exactly how I was standing, the position of my feet, the fingers of my hand, the firing of thoughts from my brain. By the end of the day I had seen that movie of my mind a thousand times. It was as though I wanted to convince myself that it was real, that it had happened that way. I also had the compulsive need to repeat it as a rite of propitiation, an offering to the goddess of fate, to convince her that I had not forgotten her touching me with the rod of death.

It was not the only mind movie I saw that day. I also watched the whole year, episode by episode, as a long narrative of my saga. Here and there, the movie lingered, describing a detail: the moment when Dr. Robbins told me that the pathologist had confirmed I had cancer; when he made me cry by asking forgiveness for taking my breast; the first meeting with the oncologist; my coming home and looking at my wounded, unibreasted chest; the meeting with the poor woman who came to the hospital at night to deliver, with sorrowful kindness, the padded acrylic breast to fill up the empty cup of my brassiere; and on and on.

When bedtime arrived, I seemed to have exhausted myself with the repeated remembrance of things past. I fell asleep and slept a dreamless night.

December 13

I could not forget. My mind insisted on remembering, day by day, the events of the previous year. It was now the time when I knew for certain that I had had an "infiltrating carcinoma, ductal and intra-ductal of the mammary gland." I knew that women my age had the worst prognosis and the highest incidence of metastasis, and that survival depended on whether there were lymph nodes involved and the nature of the treatment.

I did not have to think to know that from the depth of my soul I wanted to survive as long as I could, although my heart and my mind were filled with the gloom of death and the obscure fear of the unknown.

I remembered the frantic consultations, the running from one doctor to the other, the tests on whose results an immediate death sentence could be written in the gray ink of metastasis showing on the x-rays of my hips or lungs. Life in those ten frenetic days before the surgery was an exercise in terror and in my desperate efforts to contain it while trying to do everything that had to be done to tilt the scale of life and death in the direction of life.

I remembered with photographic memory every face that had responded for the first time to this unfamiliar, cancerous me. I remembered eyes of compassion and pathetic, furrowed foreheads, barely parted lips that exhaled words of horror and hope, restrained breathing, as though to contain a zest for life in the face of my heralded death.

I remembered the heaviness of my heart and the first details of detachment from the tree of life, like an early fall leaf beginning to dry at the base of its stem. A film of distance developed between the doer of my medicosurgical salvation and me, the cancerous woman, shaken to her foundations. I recalled watching myself come and go, listening to my doctors, going to the office to hear my patients, returning to my home; always watching myself in the act of being alive in an exercise to make believe that I could separate me, the observer, the controller, from the decay of my biological substance.

I felt again the shivering of the flesh frightened of the maiming, cutting knife, the crawling terror on the cold skin, the trembling of the lip, the moisture of the blurred eye. The gray air of remembrance and sorrow enveloped me in a winter fog for days. My eyes could not see. My senses failed to feel. I was thus frozen in reminiscence and sorrow when one Sunday morning life called me to life. My cat, Michou, had been sitting at the window for a long time, contemplating the world in front of him. An out-of-season bird flew over and, finding a branch on the tree in front of my window much to his liking and comfort, set out to give a chirping discourse on his pleasure. Michou responded with electrical excitement, meowing in an alternating duet, head out-stretched, ears pointed, tail wagging like a conductor's baton.

The air of the improvised stage vibrated with animal joy. It invited. It seduced. It tickled the skin and the senses. It opened the fallen lid to the wonders of life, not by the kiss of a prince but by the unlikely love affair of an anonymous bird and Michou, my cat. Though I was less beautiful than sleeping beauty, my eyes opened, my senses felt the gentle sting of the world's stimulation. I rubbed my eyes and my skin to inform them that they were now restored to active duty. I sat up and let all my senses open their petal-like receptors to be impregnated by all living things.

A quiet joy awoke within me while I saw the world around me: the unabashed redness of the window geraniums, their leaves competing with hues of gray and blue; the clouds puffing up their gold-rimmed bridal forms; the neighborhood houses sitting with their red brick bodies and their black slate pointed hats; a distant airplane writing its white ribbon itinerary on the sky; and Michou, his duet completed, purring and filling the air with a sea murmur.

The world lived, celebrating itself in deep color, delicate sound, mischievous shape. The world was today and always, giving a party, and the geranium and the pine tree and the cloud and the airplane and the bird and Michou and every living creature, human or beast, big or small, was invited. And so, I discovered with a smile, was I. I was invited to the party of life as long as I was alive.

How does one dress for the party of life? Does one dress in clothing or costume, makeup or natural looks? Does one respond to friends with a smile and flip answer or with the simple truth? What self does one bring to the party of life? Does one bring the one with the seven social veils or the hidden self or the bright one, dressed for the parade?

I thought that those like me, who had already met the heralds of death, should think carefully about how to go to the party of life. It was clear, as clear as the trumpets of the angels of the final day, that this was *the last party I would be invited to*, truly the last party.

December 20

The beginning of the last party began with an art festival where several of my friends were showing their years of labor, of shaping in form and color their dialogue with the world. It was a very large exhibit. Approximately 40 artists, female and male, young and old, classic and "punk" had gathered to celebrate themselves and their art. No agents or intermediaries had selected their works or imposed on them any restrictions. They had used their freedom to show themselves with bold self-acclamation, pointing to their names with bright red arrows, inviting visitors with a playful poster to come and see. They had hung bright ribbons and balloons, and those lightweight shapes danced quietly at the rhythm of a background of classical music.

My friend Adrienne, herself a part-time artist, and I went together to see what many of our mutual friends had been doing in the last three or four years in the privacy of their studios. The mood was contagious. It was all festive and joyful, like a marketplace for the arts. The place did sound like a marketplace. Unlike most exhibits, where people seem to have lost all spontaneity and have assumed solemn postures, narrowed eyes, and pursed lips in the service of showing themselves connoisseurs of "true art," here all the people seemed like children during school break. The artists in their work garments had pink cheeks and bright eyes as they welcomed their friends with kisses and hugs. Under the influence of cheese, crackers, and wine, soon everybody had pink cheeks. People spoke admiringly about a painting here and a sculpture there. Everybody was introducing everybody else. The chatting joined the background music, and the whole melange of sound appeared, to those who could enjoy it, like a phone line when the wires are crossed and one hears simultaneously many conversations and radios.

Some artists had worked on large, spectacular canvases. Others had made tiny swatches of lively creation on a square inch of surface. Some had blown glass to hues and shapes that could compete with the best displays of nature. Others had tamed clay and metal to take remarkable human and animal shapes that seemed to be waiting for the little breath of life that would allow them to move and live. Still life, living life, creature and creator, object and model, dialogue of matter and mind, of shape and texture and color, all of it was there, teeming with the tender shivering of creative birth. The midwives of beauty had filled the air with the feeling of wonder and mystery, of novelty and of the future that is reserved for witnessing a birth, the birth of the human child. Art children had been given life by many love affairs with the world.

There I was, trying to shake my fear and shivering, to have a little flirtation with the world. The work of some artists had the power to grab my spirit and get me out of myself. There was a large canvas of an opened amaryllis, unabashedly red, inviting me with casual appeal to enter the depth of its blooming petals. There was a softly colored pastel scene of three elderly people playing cards, their faces in mute dialogue with cards and friends, immersed in their pale brown atmosphere, in the simple intimacy of being there.

There was a comical metal baby, Michelinlike, made out of a bizarre mixture of ordinary tin cans, old auto parts, and a motorcycle helmet. It was a remarkably bold and unexpectedly tender little monster who, with its cold, metallic, odd shape had the power to evoke a "mother-of-the-world-to-come" affectionate smile from my lips.

There were goose-pimple-evoking pictures of horrifying Amazon snakes, green and fierce, evil eyed and fanged, arousing every unconscious fear of gigantic and destructive male organs ever dreamed of by the wildest dreamers. And there were "modern" things, good and bad, shapes so confusing that I found myself twisting my neck to invert my vision to see if I could find anything that made sense to my eyes. I did the same with some others: the odd, two-color, unshaped forms that in their defying novelty enamored the eye in spite of its rebellious resistance to their unfamiliar form.

It was all a dare, a challenge, a gentle invitation, a fierce defiance. The artists had dared to be, to create, to put into matter and on canvas the conceptions of their spirits. They had the courage to conceive their lovely and monstrous or flat-looking art children, and on top of it all, they were bragging unashamedly about them.

An obsessive doubt overcame me. I wanted to join them and laugh myself into the dance of expression and creation. But I was afraid with the fear I knew I had to live with from now on, the fear that just in the middle of the dance, when I was taken over by the exhilaration of music and fast moving legs, the music would come to an abrupt end and the loud speakers would repeat only the mournful word: metastasis . . . metastasis . . . metastasis.

I grabbed my fear by the neck as one grabs a drunkard who is obsessing with wine-filled, morbid thoughts. I was trying to bring common sense to my agitated brain. "Listen," I said to myself, "death does not send its visiting card to anybody." I was trying to quote my friend Larry when he came to console me. "You don't have to have cancer to die tomorrow in a plane crash, from an embolism or from a heart attack, or to be murdered by a dope addict. Life is always threatened. It does not come with a one- or five-year warranty. Live. Live today. Go and dance."

A popular Shakers' church melody began to play itself in my mind. I could hear every word and recall a Christmas when a choral group performed it or some Easter week when we sang it in church. Sydney Carter's lyrics went on and on in my mind:

Dance, then, wherever you may be,
I am the Lord of the dance, said he,
And I'll lead you all, wherever you may be,
And I'll lead you all in the Dance, said he.

I was absorbed in my inner listening when a deep voice said, "Hello, Madeleine, I'm so glad to see you."

I was startled. I did not expect to see him there. It was Dr. Mark Penderton, a retired professor with whom I had worked closely during my residency. We later carried out some research together and had become close and very fond of each other. I had not seen him or his wife for over a year. They had had tragedy in their lives a few years past. Their oldest daughter had died from cancer within a three-month period. At the time we all feared he could not stand the pain, and we hovered around him with respectful affection. He was a very well-loved man. I had become closer to him at the time of her illness and death.

I was overtaken by contradictory emotions. I was extremely glad to see him. We held our four hands together for a while in affectionate recognition that we had not seen each other for some time. While my hands felt the firm, strong grip of his large, bony hands, my heart was like a caged bird, fluttering wildly in my chest. I wanted to throw my arms around him, rest my head on his chest (I could never reach his tall shoulders) and sob, saying, "Mark, I had cancer." But I knew I should not do it. I did not have the right to revive the pain he was still feeling. I did not have the right to burden an elderly man with my secret.

He asked me how I was. I felt daggers in my throat when I lied and said, with my best smile, "Well, Mark, I am well, and you?" We chatted apparently freely as we had always done. I was in real pain even if I managed to cover it up. A veil separated me now, from now on, from a man I loved deeply, a man whose integrity and honesty could not be questioned; and here I was, lying through my teeth, saying that I had been too busy to call and exaggerating the number of my obligations to convince him that I had not been in touch because I had other things to do although I was really running back and forth to the hospital for dear life.

At that moment I realized that Mark was the first of some of my friends, people who were not intimate but nonetheless solid and cherished friends, who would never again fully know me. A cancer secret stood now between them and me, another pathological growth that chemotherapy could not stop. I would never again be able to give them an uncensored answer about myself. I had lost my innocence, such a precious social gift for people who could afford it.

I felt very, very sad. I could barely contain my tears after he left to see another artist's work. My dance had had an abrupt end. "Dance," I repeated, "wherever you may be," and added a verse of my own, "Dance, whatever you may feel."

December 27

A couple of weeks ago I had all my checkups. I saw three doctors, the two surgeons and my oncologist, in the span of three days. First I saw the surgeon, Dr. Robbins. He was, as usual, friendly and very open to dialogue. He was pleased with the results of his work on me. My scar was as good as a surgeon may dream it: a delicate, slightly pink line across my now apparently normal breast, stuffed with a surgical implant and crowned with a button of an insensitive nipple. He contemplated the work of his colleague, Dr. Keily, the plastic surgeon. "Dr. Keily," he said with genuine admiration, "has done a great job." I agreed. I could, if I wanted, wear anything and, perhaps, nobody could tell I had had a mastectomy. My breasts seemed practically equal in size and were indistinguishable to the eye. Touching them was another matter. Normal breast tissue, with its tender softness had been replaced on my right side by a more rubbery substance, firm and unfeeling. The whole skin surface of the breast had only a dull capacity for sensation and response. The back of my arm and the area around the back of my shoulder were also dull. A whole year had now gone by, and Dr. Robbins and I acknowledged to each other that I would never recover normal sensitivity in those areas of my body. The contemplation of my reconstructed breast completed, Dr. Robbins proceeded to examine my other breast. He has a very expressive face. A cloud of gloom passed over his hazel eyes, and a wave of sorrow sat on his well-formed lips. His hands examined my left breast, asking questions of every millimeter of breast tissue under my skin. They touched lightly, pushed, compressed, touched again and then slid to the axillary pit, searching for lymph nodes. Finally they crossed my middle and went to the base of my neck on the other side, and the axillary pit, this time searching for potential metastatic lymph nodes. A deep, dense silence involved the dialogue of his hands with my body. Finally he smiled broadly and said triumphantly, "I don't find anything. It seems to me you are very well."

He asked me if I felt well. I laughed and said that I felt so well that I had decided to live to 88. Dr. Robbins became pale, leaned forward, and said with undisguised horror, "But we are in '88!" It took me a second to see what had happened. Dr. Robbins thought I had said I was not going to live beyond 1988, and it was now January 1988. I laughed again and said as fast as I could, "Oh, no, no! I have no intention of dying. I mean I am going to live *until* I am 88 years old, like most people in my family." This time he blushed. We both understood what had happened but preferred not to make it explicit. Dr. Robbins, from the beginning of my cancer diagnosis, had thought that the chances of my having metastases and cancer in the other breast were pretty high and that there was a need to monitor my health very carefully because my prognosis was not as good as statistics said it should be. It was clear that he was concerned about my survival. I was of two hearts. It warmed me to see that he cared deeply about me. It scared me that he seemed to have me scheduled for an earlier death than he himself would like.

We chatted for a while, making believe that nothing had happened. He always addressed me as a colleague and let me say my part as explicitly as I wanted. He said he wanted blood tests and a mammogram. It had been 20 months since the last one, the one where cancer was not found, even when by hindsight one could detect it in the film. I said that Dr. Nagle was going to do all that in a few days and that it did not make sense to me to duplicate the tests. He agreed and charged me with the message to Dr. Nagle that he wanted copies of the lab results and of the mammogram report. I promised to fulfill my messenger's task.

He then looked at me for a final appraisal of all of me. "You look very well," he said with obvious satisfaction.

"I feel very well," I said, "I still have to lose the pounds I gained with the chemotherapy. Then I'll be myself again." He asked if I was dieting. I said I was only eating a little less and exercising as much as I could. He approved of it. He asked me to return in six months and again expressed his pleasure at seeing me and seeing me looking and feeling well.

I left feeling that he was truly a good and competent man who cared for me. I found myself thinking that I would probably see him a couple of more times, and then he would go out of my life, to enter the lives of others as he had entered mine, carrying with his presence the double message of surgical pain and bad tidings and of his kind and caring dedication to the task. I had grown very fond of him, and I knew I was going to miss him when my checkups were completed.

Soon after, I went to the plastic surgeon. He was in an unusually good mood, and his voice had a warbler's song in it. He asked me how I was and if I was having any problem with the implant. I told him I was feeling very well, finally, and that the implant was doing well under my skin. A minor skin rash still persisted near the surgical wound, but that was all, a little bit of itching.

He asked me to disrobe, danced out of the room, and returned in a few minutes with a knock on the door asking if I was ready. For reasons I do not know, his nurse was not there. He came in, examined me very carefully, checking everything thoroughly: the site of the stitches, the consistency of the implant, the probable formation of a "capsule" around it, the site where the "port" had been.

He explained that everything was progressing normally and that the skin rash was probably due to an abnormal skin reaction to the catgut used for stitching but there was nothing to worry about. The implant would become softer with time. The port had caused the tissue around it to form a little channel to contain it. It would take months for it to be reabsorbed. At this point, Dr. Keily entered his fascinating surgical world. His eyes turned dreamy while he described with excitement how shiny and pretty and beautiful this little cavity, the skin made for the port, was. One could see him looking with his surgical magnifying lenses into that little body cavity that so fascinated him. I said sympathetically that I could imagine how pretty it was, but I now told my side of the story, that I was going to be pleased if that fascinating "lump" on top of my ribs went away. I reminded myself of the famous phrase of the French scientist Lecomte du Noüy, "The point of view creates the phenomenon." He reassured me that it would be gone in six months.

It was clear that he could do two things at once. He was obviously talking to me, but his eyes were still having "fun" with the little shiny cavity. His hands, placed in front of him, clasped the folder with my record. At that moment he went through his looking glass and entered the wonderland of his beloved plastic surgery. He stood there motionless, his eyes fixed on my breasts, very slowly going from the normal to the repaired breast. He contemplated, operated, reflected, corrected, imagined, all silently for a long time. Slowly the eyes traveled from the depth of the breast tissue to the surface of the skin. His eyes darted faster from breast to breast and slowly, like the sun rising in a clear morning, a smile illuminated his face until, it broke into the self-congratulatory words, "It looks good to me."

"You did a magnificent job," I said. "I am very grateful to you now that I am double-breasted again." He laughed. "It makes a great difference," I said. "I feel free again, normal again." He smiled. "I still have to lose some weight. I lost a little."

"You look very trim," he said with a remote, dreamy voice. He was neither thinking about me nor looking at me any longer. He had reentered the dream world of surgery. He stayed there for a while. I could see that he was seeing things I could not see. Finally he came out of it and said a bit embarrassedly, "You can get dressed. I don't need you undressed." He did not, however, feel too repentant about having gone off into his dream world, and I was not upset by his behavior. Indeed I liked him for it. He was one of the very few men of his age, in his middle fifties, still capable of experiencing the total fascination of a child. He had made a profession of it, a private world, a marvelous universe of beautiful shapes and glittering surfaces. I was secretly proud that in my maimed condition I could offer him beautiful tissues to contemplate and play with.

Having returned to the world of human commerce, he asked me if I needed anything. I said no, and he wished me well and said he wanted to see me in six months. As I had with Dr. Robbins, I had grown very, very fond of this competent and mature man who could become a marvelously playful child at the snap of a finger. Secretly I harbored the hope that perhaps I would have to see him every so often even though I could not be sure what for. I had forgiven him for the mess he had made of the date of the surgery, the way one forgives a bright child who gets all excited with his toys. I had come to see that it was not malice but his irrepressible trips to the wonderland of surgical glitter that made him forget the obvious practicalities of life.

January 3

My next visit was to the oncologist. Dr. Nagle was a half hour late, as was customary in his clinic. The patients, in various states of cancerous deterioration, helped themselves to coffee and read magazines. Others, too weak to do anything, sat, their eyes lost in a remote vision. Some were in wheelchairs with nurse practitioners next to them to carry them around.

I sat in the most hidden corner, afraid, as I always was, to be seen by some colleague or former student who knew me.

The nurse, a large, deep-voiced, black woman, read aloud my first name. In those circumstances I had given up my protest about being called by my first name, something I would not tolerate in a private office. It annoys me that men are called Mister X or Z, while I am called Madeleine by a woman barely out of her teens. I always make a fuss, ask her to read the M.D. on my chart, and request that she call me Dr. Meldin, as she would if I were a male doctor. This time I had neither the wish to fight for the respect due the female gender nor the need to make myself conspicuous, a cancerous object.

I followed the nurse. She weighed me and congratulated me for having lost seven of the 13 pounds I had gained with the chemotherapy. My blood pressure was slightly high. She measured it three times, and it dropped a bit. Obviously I was more anxious than I was willing to admit to myself.

Dr. Nagle came in with his usual quiet smile and half-comical eyebrow signals. He congratulated me on my weight loss and asked me about my general condition. I said I was feeling so well that I had decided to return to my original life plan and join my family in living to my 88th year. He looked at me and purposely making a face of great surprise asked, "Why so young?"

"That is my plan," I said firmly.

"Fine," he said. "Then I can examine you."

He seemed to be asking to be part of my survival program. He dashed out of the room, and I changed into a striped white and green robe—a new design for the patient's elegance—and produced my personal illness notebook with a list of all we had to discuss in this consultation.

He returned and examined me, searching for lumps on the normal breast and lymph nodes everywhere. I was clear of any symptom. He looked at my breasts and said with genuine admiration, "Dr. Keily did a fantastic job. Your breasts look terrific." I agreed and said that I was very pleased and very grateful for the help I had been given.

He asked me to dress again and, with a vigorous gesture, drew the curtain between his desk and the examining table so he could write his notes and I could dress. He asked from the other side of the curtain, "What do you have in your notebook?" I told him about a couple of prescriptions I needed. He wrote them up while I finished dressing. We seemed to be well synchronized. I drew the curtain out of the way at the moment he was signing the second prescription.

We then went over the list. We discussed flu vaccination; I would get it at once. Next, we spoke about exercise and weight loss. He agreed that I was doing what I was supposed to. With regard to checkups, today he was going to give me a battery of blood tests, and, if everything was normal, I did not have to see him for four months. He wanted me to go for a mammogram to an excellent breast clinic where they examine you very carefully and give you the results before you leave. He gave me the number to call for the appointment. I told him that Dr. Robbins, the surgeon, wanted the reports of the blood tests and the mammogram. He promised to send them along.

Now the moment had come for the question that needed to be answered a million times: prognosis. He repeated himself. I would probably be free of metastasis for five or ten years. Everything had gone well so far.

"Those are statistics," I said, talking to him and to myself, "and I have to make peace with my own death, whatever way it comes. I have to prepare myself for both: for a long life and for a death that may come sooner than I like." He agreed. He asked me about my relatives in remote parts of the world. It was clear that he had something in mind. Soon he said it, as though he wanted to make sure that I was carrying out well my preparation for death.

"Most of the people who die of cancer regret not having been close to their families while there was still time."

I understood immediately what he meant. He was directly addressing my situation as a woman alone, who would die alone, without relatives around even when I had many very faithful friends. I understood that he knew the business of the human heart at the final hour of death. He wanted me to use any time I had, brief or long, to stretch out a friendly hand to my alienated relatives.

I was moved and frightened, fearful of my inability to bring my efforts to any level of meaningful human communication. I was wary of the hidden resentments in the dark recesses of my heart, of the wish to reject *them*, of the need to "show them."

"Forgiveness," I said humbly, "is the most difficult thing in the world. I am trying, and I need all the help I can get, from dialogue and support to prayers. I need a lot of help. If I continue to do well, I shall go soon to see my relatives. I'll try the best I can to compensate for the bitterness of being unable to have a dialogue with those who are of my own blood."

"Family, family," he chuckled.

I could not pick up his modulating ironic mood. I was hurting too much. I kept going on with what I had to say to myself in the first place.

"I am examining, and I will continue to examine, what part I may have in this alienation. It is very difficult to be objective. I am trying my best to look at our family history from the point of view of my relatives. I know you are right. I am trying the best I can, although I fear my best is not good enough."

He said nothing but smiled sympathetically. After a few seconds he said, "I'll get Monique to give you the flu shot. I want to see you in four months. Take care." He left, and I stayed in the consulting room. Monique came in, shining like the spring sun. She had photographs in her hands. She greeted me very warmly, fussed about my looking healthy, and without undue delay showed me the pictures of her baby. She had delivered her five or six days after she gave me my last dose of chemotherapy. I was the last patient she saw before her maternity leave.

The baby, smiling and bright eyed, sat on her little chair showing the world that she felt herself the queen of the universe. All of her shone with excitement and life. Her mother was celebration itself. Obviously those two were having a tremendous love affair, a continuous echo of mutual admiration, a song duet, celebrating themselves. I too fell under the spell of the baby's picture and began praising mother and child with great enthusiasm. Monique seemed to have a moment of self-consciousness and said, "My husband too is crazy about her. He is a basket case. She adores him." One could see "the family," the glorious beginning of a new life, the bringing to existence a child of love. One could see the enormous seductiveness of a brand new infant.

"The family," I reflected sadly to myself, "before the original sin, before misunderstanding, rivalry, hatred, unrequited love."

There is wisdom, I felt, in a baby's irresistible charm. It is that bond, those memories of shining eyes, of playful mouths, of excited bodies, of dialogues without words that bond us forever to each other and give us the hope that human communication is possible, always possible.

Monique could not stop talking about Kate, her baby. She went on and on about every little thing the child did, had done, or would do. Finally she said laughingly, "I'd better give you the flu shot." Under the spell of Kate, the newborn queen, we went with light hearts and light feet to the nurses' station.

We said good-bye. I had my blood drawn by another nurse and made an appointment for the mammogram.

I went to the radiology department for the mammogram after a fitful night. I could not sleep. I did not want to admit to myself how frightened I was. Dr. Robbins had said explicitly that he was worried that I would develop cancer in my other breast and had urged me to have the mammogram as soon as possible. Dr. Nagle had disagreed. Fear, however, sticks to gloomy forecasts, and I was afraid. I had flashes of a moment when the radiologist would say that I had a lump on the other breast. Then I could feel my world collapsing again. I fantasized another mastectomy, more plastic surgery, another six months of chemotherapy. I felt a tremendous sense of oppression and despair, as though the universe had no air left for me to breathe. I tried to be as brave as I could, to be ready for bad news. It was easy to be ready for good news. Freedom and joy would then come my way. It was horrifying to prepare for bad news. I could feel the wish to give up, to surrender to death, to let the rotten flesh rot the rest of me. So in between hope and fear, I slept and woke up a thousand times that night before the mammogram.

The radiologist's office, located in a corner of the huge hospital complex, was pleasant, had flowers in the waiting room and a relaxed atmosphere. The nurse was efficiency in person. We settled our business, and I waited for a few moments. A nurse wearing an x-ray apron called *my last name* (never a good sign) and took me to a little room with lockers. She asked me to "take everything off from the waist up" and then to wait in the second waiting room. There I met my fellow patients. I felt ashamed when I caught myself staring, one by one, at their breasts to see if they, as I had, had lost a breast. I was an expert now. I could tell the difference between a natural breast and an implant or a reconstructed breast. A real breast has the natural protruding elegance of living things pushing forward. Plastic surgery breasts are a presence on a chest, a body of mounting flesh without a living voice. A trained eye, sharp and searching, could tell the difference between breasts covered by only the thin layer of the examining gown. There were four women there. Two were in their early 40s and two in their 60s. My eye saw that their breasts, hanging down from their chests like ripe soft fruits on a summer tree, had descended a little in their downward way to aging and moved with their owners' movements with gelatinlike waves of healthy flesh. I laughed secretly, feeling like a lecherous man or a lesbian hopelessly fixed on breasts' attractions.

The nurse with the apron came to get me. She talked in a matter-of-fact way about my cancer. I told her about the location of the cancer in my removed breast. She was very careful trying to get a perfect view. It was clear that she was proud of her work and eager to do it well. She sent me back to the waiting room. In less than ten minutes another nurse came in saying that Dr. Nyman, the radiologist, wanted to show me the x-rays. Dr. Nyman, a very pleasant man, stood up, shook my hand, and welcomed me as a colleague. Without waiting a second he showed me the x-rays and said that I was perfectly well. There was no sign of any lesion, cancerous or not. Technically, I could see that the x-rays were of excellent quality. Every detail was clearly visible. He was looking at them with a huge magnifying glass. He invited me to look and explained a few things. We talked then about the unusual location of my cancer. He said that for our, his and my, peace of mind he was going to ask the technician to take a special view of the axillary area. I was relieved and grateful for his openness. I returned to the waiting room. New women had replaced my former companions. I did not check their breasts. The technician fetched me again, took the new view, and developed the film. I was back with Dr. Nyman, who said triumphantly, "Dr. Meldin, you are perfectly well. There is nothing abnormal in your breast. You need not return for a year." I felt an immense gratitude toward him as though he had performed the miracle of curing me of the many cancers my imagination had developed in my breasts.

7

Making Peace

January 17

I now had a "medical vacation." After running to doctors, tests, and x-rays for more than a year, I had, for the first time since the discovery of the lump, four months without any medical appointments. My life was beginning to return to its normal, well-scheduled, disciplined pace. Perhaps it was time to resume all that had been interrupted by the cancer. Perhaps I should call the travel agent and find an excursion to a warm climate or maybe return to the original plan of visiting the Caribbean. I did have some good friends there, people I had met through my activities in different conferences and professional meetings. Or I could go to visit my relatives and try to get some conversation, some dialogue going with them. The beauty of it all was that I could do any of those things, that my life, now free of threatening death, was mine again, and I could use it, live it, enjoy it, celebrate it.

My body too had recovered its balance. I could feel it healthy. My limbs were no longer heavy and disinclined to move. My skin had returned to a subtle pinky, shiny hue. My eyelids were no longer heavy. My muscles had a natural disposition to movement, like those of a well-trained horse waiting for a light signal to trot here or there. Nimble is the word for it. My body, heavy and burdened for over a year, had become nimble, rhythmical again, attuned to the cosmic music of the spheres. It wanted to dance the dance of life.

One evening, while thinking these thoughts and feeling these marvelous bodily feelings, I decided to have a little private celebration. I played on the tape deck the spring music of Vivaldi's *Four Seasons*. I took off my shoes, and fancying myself a spring fairy or a prima ballerina or both, I let the joy of my body create its own choreography.

Michou, my cat, seemed to understand what it was all about. He dashed back and forth from one corner of the living room to the other, suddenly stopped at the center, mewed dramatically, jumped to the window, made a pirouette, descended to the couch, rested for a minute and then, excited again, ran around the room, following my steps. We made a fine, if odd, dancing pair. I stopped, exhausted, and sat in the middle of the rug. Michou took his place on the couch with recovered dignity, his white-gloved paws outstretched, and contemplated me with questioning eyes.

"Michou," I said in response, "life is a wonderful gift, a joyous present. You and I are going to celebrate it everyday, in our little ways. We are going to enjoy the sun, the air, our friends, the birds, the plants in the house, our food, the gift of water (that maternal and tender creature). We are going to listen for the little voices of all living creatures. We are going to sing with them. We are going to tell all our friends that life is a dance and ask them to dance with us. Yes, Michou, that is what we are going to do. I mean what *I* am going to do. I have seen you doing it when you get so excited with the birds and so happy with caresses and food. I am joining you."

Michou looked at me intently all the time while I delivered my solemn speech to him. When I finished, he stretched out, front paws down, rear end up, and descended from the couch like the king of the jungle from a mountain top. He stopped in front of me and meowed. I knew that he wanted me to pick him up and tickle his head a little. I did, and he began a contented purring concert, directed by his wagging tail. It was all made to measure: a concerto harmonicus of Michou and myself, content and joyful with our living friendship.

That was, at least for the time being, the end of my illness. I was, in fact, free of cancer. It could recur anytime. Or it might never reappear again. I was once more like all women, men, children, animals or plants: a normally fragile, living being. Death, the terminator, could meet me and any of us, unsuspecting, or it could send its visiting card announcing its imminent visitation. I was no longer the one "marked for death." I had been removed from death row and placed back among the common folk. I felt a gratitude so deep that I am not sure I can fully express it.

I was grateful to my body in the first place. My gratitude was colored by a sense of awe, the same awe I had experienced when I studied medicine and discovered the perfection, the complexity, the elegance of the body as architecture and as functions. Now I was grateful for the faithfulness, the awesome faithfulness of my body, not only for providing me with this very enjoyable feeling of well-being but also for returning to its prechemotherapy shape. I felt like calling the spirit of Walt Whitman to ask him to help me write a new ad hoc *Song of Myself,* celebrating the recovery of a well tuned clavier, my body.

I also felt intense gratitude to all the branches of the medical sciences. I knew that as recently as 50 years ago my only prognosis would have been a slow or rapid progress to a metastatic death. The fact that I had a chance for a cancer-free life was the result of innumerable hours of research, exploration, experimentation, writing, presenting papers in congresses, comparing ideas, arguing, experimenting again, and researching some more – the work of thousands of practitioners and scientists of many disciplines.

I wished I could send a little card to all those still alive and put a flower on the graves of those who were dead who had contributed to my rescue.

I wanted to thank all the clinicians of the past 50 years who strained themselves and their thought processes to find better ways to help women with breast cancer.

I wanted to thank all the surgeons and plastic surgeons who (like Dr. Keily) in their mental surgeries imagined new ways to tame their scalpels so that they could heal with minimal injury. I wanted to thank them for all the papers they wrote, all the discussions they participated in, all the congresses they attended to learn how to help us.

I wanted to thank all the chemists, biologists, pathologists, and cell researchers for their efforts to find drugs to heal us and methods to diagnose our cancer better. I wanted to thank them for the endless hours of patient work, so often without any results or any glory for so much effort. I wanted to thank their humble rats and mice, which were called to duty without consent and offered their pain and their small lives in the service of our future salvation. I wanted to thank

them, all those unnamed little female creatures who developed horrible, man-inflicted mammary cancers and died of them so that we
could live. I asked their forgiveness for having suffered so that my
sisters and I could live.

I wanted to thank all the members of surgical teams, from surgeon
and anesthesiologist to scrub nurses and engineers, who design operating room equipment. All their joint efforts had greatly contributed
to my going through surgery three times with minimal pain and
excellent results.

I wanted to thank all the nurses, secretaries, and attendants who,
by being there at their jobs each day, had made possible the chain of
events that permitted me to go from being a woman with a breast
invaded by cancer to being a woman with a body free of cancer.

I wanted to thank nature itself and her Maker, because hidden in
the heart of matter there are mysterious chemicals and unexpected
molecules waiting to be called to duty by scientific discovery to fulfill
their healing potential.

My lengthy act of gratitude brought new awareness. I had never
realized how interdependent people and things are on one another.
Suddenly the words of Ernesto Cardenal came to mind:

> To keep the cycle of life going we feed on each other, we literally, we all
> living beings, eat each other up. We grow to feed others and others
> before us have grown to feed us. The tiger eats the gazelle, the gazelle
> eats the grass, the grass feeds on the remnants of living things of the
> past, the living things of the past were forest and birds and dinosaurs
> and tigers of sorts. A cycle – life is a cycle, and we are all to be recycled.

I felt a communication with all living things and a strange and
amusing pleasure at the thought that my precious little body was made
out of recycled elements, recombined atoms that had had their share
of reincarnations. I found myself laughing with good-hearted amazement. I had never had these thoughts before. It felt good to have them.
It was like belonging to a kingdom, a country, a community. I
remembered that as a child of seven when I was introduced to zoology
and "the animal kingdom" I was very impressed that all animals
belonged to the same kingdom while we humans had so many nations
that I could not count them on my school map. "Good," I said now,
"good. All living things belong to the kingdom of life." This I said in all

seriousness and with great pleasure now, when my age was eight times seven.

Encouraged by these thoughts, I decided to look again at the chain of events started by my discovering I had cancer. "In what way," I asked myself, "do we need each other, we who were involved in my year's journey through the land of the deadly enemy?" I discovered that if we, the cancerous ones, did not have cancer, my oncologist would have had to change his specialty, my surgeon would have had fewer patients to operate on, and the plastic surgeon would not have been able to make mud pies on women's chests. The scientists would have had to research something else, and we all would have had to change.

It would have been better if we could eradicate cancer, but we have not done it yet. So, for the time being, we were like links on a chain, holding each other in a circle of events. Our lives were interdependent. To eat, literally, to earn their money, they needed us. To survive, to be able to keep eating, we, the cancerous ones, needed them.

A good feeling came upon me. Used to the Protestant ethic of our nation, we have grown individualistic, self-sufficient, and righteous; we have a feeling of entitlement and demanding what is our due. It is to our benefit that we have done so. Justice, equality, and respect are democratic virtues as fragile as our lives. Constant vigilance is needed to keep them alive and in force. Each citizen is responsible for keeping them alive and working in her or his life. The struggle, however, should not make us forget, as I had until this rude awakening, that vigilance is not enough. Beyond that is the need we all have for each other, the way in which our lives are enmeshed and intertwined, the sick feeding the healthy and the healthy nurturing the sick. I had now experienced both aspects. I had just emerged from the ranks of the sick and rejoined the healthy.

I had to get used to being healthy again. I was pulled equally by hope and by fear. On the side of hope, I wanted to fully return to life, to all my activities, to work, to commitments, to friends. I wanted to cook, to travel, to pot and unpot my plants, to play with Michou, to visit with friends, to see if I could make contact with some blood relative, to go to the movies, to plays, to concerts, to attend church, to walk around, to laugh, to talk silly, to dream and daydream, to let myself go with the whole flow of the waters of life.

On the side of fear, there was a trembling in my flesh, an unnamed horror for the potential metastatic cell that could announce its presence just when I was in the middle of laughter and bring my joy of living to a screeching halt.

I realized that I had to make peace with both possibilities. To be able to live fully, I had to be willing to die when death came for me; I had to count death not as an enemy, a robber, or a deceiver. I had to accept that I was mortal like all creatures. Life was not something due me. Life is a gift, a very generous gift. If I was willing to enjoy it, I had to be willing to give it back when my turn came, as all living beings have done since the beginning of time. I had to accept my own recycling if I wanted to take part in the cycle. I found peace in thinking about fruits, so delicious and refreshing. Their highest achievement, their succulent ripeness comes at the end of their cycle, the best moment for surrendering their lives.

"Perhaps," I thought, trying to be very brave, "I should be like a fruit the gardener did not pick at the time of the last crop, a fruit that was given time to ripen, to enhance its flavor. I'm old enough, and it's time for me to ripen. This cancer had given me a message. I'd better hurry up in case I have to go soon. It would not be right to be a bitter fruit at the moment I was picked from the tree of life."

The voice said, "Well, well, see how far you have come now. Be glad. You are like fruit, like wine. You have time to enhance your flavor, to age gracefully until you become mellow and delicate to yourself and others."

The gift of the life I had left, short or long, was in my hands. I could live it with joy and celebration and with just a bit of fear and trembling while I still had it.

I did not think I needed a lesson in living. My encounter with cancer had taught me a lesson in humility, though. I had learned, in my very flesh, about my own mortality and that of all human beings. I had learned about our (sometimes unwilling) solidarity with one another and with the whole of nature.

I had discovered that we can get so immersed in our everyday lives that we forget how precious life itself is. I had found that the smallest of things counts, that Michou's enthusiasm for a bird is not less important than the ecstasy of a lover or a beautiful operatic aria. All things, big and small, count, every smile and every tear. Simply to appreciate what is there now is what life is all about. Simply to appreciate the riches in the temporal stream of our personal lives may be the deepest act of thanksgiving we can offer to the Giver of all Life.

This is what I learned when I came out of my dark night of cancerous illness.

Epilogue

Four years have passed since the moment when an unsuspecting finger met the cancerous grain in my breast. For cancer patients, the number four evokes feelings that oscillate between gratitude for survival and fear of hoping. It is one digit removed from the magical five, the marker of the first statistical bend for survivors who may go on to the next turn, ten years. Each new period of time after finding and the immediate treatment of the cancer brings with it complex feelings, contradictory wishes, paradoxical responses to the simple realities of everyday life. A comparison to the experience of combat veterans is not only apt but also accurate. There are flashbacks to the moments of maximum horror; there are feelings of not being quite there in the world of the normally living; there is a sense of having come back, like a Vietnam veteran, from a remote and bewildering reality without feeling any pride in the wounds left by a war. To reenter my everyday life, I, the cancer patient, had to force myself to identify my very complex feelings as a way of confronting the obscure rattlings and rumblings in the background of each of my experiences. The sounds enwrapped me in a melancholic cloud, a mournful mood, at times soft and gentle, at other times suffocating.

The first six months after all surgery and treatments had been completed, I had a *bodily* feeling that I had to inform myself that I existed in a real reality. There was no psychopathology in this, but the feeling of wonder and of distorted recognition one experiences when returning for the first time to a well-remembered childhood dwelling. The eyes of the eight-year-old child saw it from the child's height, a few inches lower than the revisiting adult. The picture of the Chinese dragon on the wall, once so terrifying, has become a plain silver beast on a red background. The high ceiling has descended a few feet; the room has become smaller. It is the same room, and the feelings of recognition and the memories rush to the heart. Yet it is not the same room. The adult brings to it a different perspective, a paradoxical recognition of what was there, unseen before: the photograph of the elegant grandfather, now dead; the parental diploma never read.

My body was at the beginning of its return, as old as it was new. My senses had acquired a new acuity, a keenness for detail and form, for meaning and message. I attended to reality, internal and external, with eager curiosity, instinctual and searching, rising from the lost pilgrim's anguish in the dark forest. The experience called for a remapping of the whole world, finding new paths to climb to the fullness of life. Simple exchanges with people acquired unsuspected dimensions: a clerk's smile in a store seemed like a gift, a child's cry felt like choral confirmation of universal pain, a firm handshake a proof of living bodies in warm contact. Everything had the newness of what is refound in a new key, a sort of symphonic transformation of well known tunes.

My reaction amazed me. After all, I had not left the world. My hospitalizations for the mastectomy and the plastic surgery had been brief. I had not stopped working, although I had reduced my schedule to a much lighter load. I kept in contact with my friends, read the papers, listened to the radio, watched the news, and participated in the usual passions of public events. Why, then, was I experiencing the world as though I had just returned from a remote galaxy? The world had not changed because I had had cancer. It had to be I who had changed. In what way? In what manner? After much self-scrutiny, I realized that my point of view had changed. I had been used to taking life, people, the world for granted. The world, sure enough, could still be taken for granted, but I could not take myself for granted. I had become aware, not without resentful indignation at first and humble acceptance later, that I was dispensable, the world could do without me. Humbled by my superfluous existence, I felt the need to recarve a niche for myself. It was clear that I had not lost my concrete position in the world. The niche I am talking about has to do with the ethereal space where the act of being takes place, that imperceptible region more real than the space occupied by bodies.

It all happened as though I had to learn anew everything I knew and that I had never forgotten. I found myself absorbed in thought, contemplating the simplest and most pedestrian events: the street lights blinking in dutiful succession – red, yellow, green, red, yellow, green – like a city heart beating, like my heart beating – for how long? When would the electricity stop, the machinery fail . . . red, yellow, green, red. . . . I crossed the street with the solemnity of a soul crossing Acheron.

On the other side of the street awaited a splendid shop. In its windows, wide-eyed, slim, sexual, and distantly enticing mannequins dressed in high-fashion evening clothes displayed their fixed beauty. I was transfixed, and before I knew it – I had lost many of the pounds I had gained with the chemotherapy – I was trying on a black and red dress that made me look like a young and desirable woman capable of astonishing some well-known gentlemen who would never have imagined me so fancy a dresser. It was all new, as though I had never had had an elegant dress wrapping my not unattractive figure. The difference was in the feeling. There was a new joy there, the natural joy of the imagined new "me" shockingly "beautiful." And so I went like a blind person who has been given sight, looking at everything, inhaling life everywhere.

The intensity of this looking and inhaling the whole world continued for the whole of the first year after my recovery. Then it blended progressively with other thoughts and feelings but never disappeared completely. It became a soft note, a delicate humming, a musical commentary to my feelings about the astonishing act of living.

While I was going from surprise to surprise, I still had my body to attend to. My medical body, my personal body, both me's in my body. The doctors had spoken gently but firmly about my medical body. I needed rigorous follow-up for several years. I was to be attentive for any signs of metastatic illness. I was to watch out for osteoporosis because I could not take any hormones. Extra milk and calcium plus exercise had to be part of my regimen. I had to examine my other breast carefully and frequently. I had to take care of the gynecological consequences of having no sexual hormones in circulation, in particular of vaginal changes. I was to be very careful not to injure the arm on the side of the mastectomy because many lymph nodes had been removed, and there was a risk of infection. I was not to have blood drawn from that arm. Finally, I had to protect my "breast implant" (such a botanical term!) from being punctured, and therefore deflated, and losing its form-enhancing shape.

The warnings were reasonable and relatively simple. My feelings about them were complex: a mixture of a sensation of being made of fragile porcelain and of having to keep the watchfulness of a jealous dog. And with them was fear, deep, all encompassing, irrational, reasonable; the fear was always there. Each morning brought with my early shower the panic about my fingers' potential new "encounters." Each visit to the oncologist and the surgeon every three months was a horrible ordeal of terror. The conviction that he would find a new node, a metastasis, preceded each visit. The oncologist's respectful humor and the surgeon's cheerful disposition dispelled the "certainty" that they would find a new cancerous growth only at the last minute of the visit. Besides, I developed innumerable "metastases" on my own. Each bone, head, or muscle ache became a metastasis. I developed a trick to calm myself down: I ordered myself to wait three days, "which would not aggravate any existing metastasis," before I called the doctor. I was "cured" of all of them except one which was "healed" by negative x-rays. Happily, I remained in excellent health, and the weight of reality calmed me down, but not completely. I still worry each time I go to see the oncologist or when I experience an unrecognizable pain.

The preoccupation with my medical body was constant. At first no hour went by without my having some thought about "my" cancer. Disbelief, horror, watchfulness, predictions, anticipation, double checking, reviewing to the last comma each medical conversation, each medical article, each reference to prognostic clues were activities that went on like a merry-go-round that I could not control. As time passed, the turning and churning of thoughts and worries slowed down bit by bit until finally, one day late in my third year after the event, I realized that I had gone through the entire day without thinking about cancer. It was like becoming free again or, rather, like being on probation, because many days followed when I returned to my slow turning of concerns. I do not believe it is possible to be completely free from worry. Cancer is a treacherous tenant unwilling to leave the premises it once inhabited. To watch out for its return may be nerve wracking but life saving. Wisdom, for the lucky ones who attain it, lies in between these two extremes.

Nor was personal body easier to handle than my medical body. I became something that I can only call a "self-voyeur." I was constantly looking at myself out of the corner of my eye in window shops, in mirrors, and in the reflected response of the eyes of others looking at me. I was always checking to see if my dark secret, my fake breast, showed through my visible figure. Seeing a shapely enough and unrevealing reflection did not cure my half-paranoid conviction that "they" could see that my breasts were not exactly alike. My certified anatomical knowledge that all women have uneven breasts made no impression on me. There was in my rejection of the objective fact a subjective truth. My sensory nerves performed their informative task with accurate precision: they told me that I had one breast that had the natural weight and suppleness of healthy human flesh, and another that was rubbery, heavy, and dead under the concealing skin. Whether I sat or walked, lay down, or stood up, the nerves insisted on repeating the same asymmetric messages. They also persisted in informing me that the rest of me was perfectly symmetrical.

Choosing clothes and brassieres became a difficult task. My surgically repaired breast was slightly smaller than the other and did not have the normal forwardness (as the plastic surgeon described it) of the other breast. The brassiere had to perform that task for it. After much searching and rehearsing, I finally settled for a particular type of garment that offered firm support to both breasts. As for clothes, I was inclined to dress like an old-fashioned nun, so wrapped in fabric that you may wonder whether there is a body there. It was only through progressive, small acts of courage, one dress at a time, that I returned to the tailored clothes more suited to my figure. Each new transformation back to my former body shape was followed by self-voyeuristic episodes and suspicious moods.

There still remained my naked body to deal with. There was no deception. The sensory nerves and my well-informed eyes converged in sad agreement. The plastic surgeon had provided the best substitute his technical skill could offer. A good breast for sartorial satisfaction, for sculptural symmetry, but no more. Sitting on my rib cage, entrapped there in the pectoral muscle, was that soft, inert mass pretending to be a breast, under a barely alive skin of deadened sensibility and crowned by a button of knotted flesh imitating, with irritating unselfconsciousness, a milk fountain, an exquisite bud for sexual awakening.

I and my body knew the absence of dialogue between bodies lay in my muted breast. We knew the shame of unresponsiveness to embrace and touch, to the pressing of bodies asking flesh questions to be answered in reflexive delight. Each prospective embrace became shameful anticipation, until I could pull my self up to the level of memory capable of recalling that affection and love cut deeper than the lack of reflexes of dead flesh. The true affection of those who loved me, and their freedom to be spontaneous and physical with me, convinced me beyond doubt that I was bigger than my breast. The lesson, however, had been a painful one, for at my worst moments I came close to believing that I was less than my implanted breast. Finally, after much effort at self-acceptance, I came to see that the person who was the last to accept me as I was now was I. In a conscious confrontation with myself, I stood naked in front of the mirror and carried out aloud my accepting act: "This is you now, as you are"—I said to my image—"a healed, wounded body, keeping you as you always were." I must have understood myself, because I felt at peace.

Slowly, one feeling at a time, my life reentered its previous automatic mode. Going to gatherings no longer held the constant danger of a self-betraying body or the previous acute pain of meeting friends who knew nothing about my having been ill. Normal psychic repression resumed its very helpful function, and I could now do most of what I wanted to do without going through the ordeal of an emotional storm. Approximately at the end of the second year, a new mood came over me, a contemplative mood far removed from the one of bewildered looking at the blinking street lights. I began to look at life in its broadest aspects. In a mellow and tender mood, I found myself pondering little Michou's life: his cat beauty, his softness, his constant search to be close to me and to play with whatever and whomever he found in his path. I found it wondrous that six pounds of flesh and fur, allotted a maximum of 16 years of earthly enjoyment, could be so simply joyful and so profoundly meaningful to me and to his many human and nonhuman friends.

I looked at seeds, grains of life, and I witnessed their amazing transformation into plants a million times the original size. I read about some paleobotanists who had brought to germination seeds of grain that had been waiting for 2,000 years to sprout. Called to life, the seeds pushed aside their ancient coats, and the grains became normal plants. Fruit, dormant for two millenia, graced their branches.

These are just small samples of my many contemplative thoughts. Something was dawning on me, a new way of looking at the whole phenomenon of life, beyond individuals and generations. It was not a thought, but a feeling of solidarity, of continuity, of the paradox of the unique value of each individual life and its limited but indispensable participation with a long chain of interconnected creatures from the beginning of time, through now, on the way to tomorrow. I laughed when I became fully aware of my way of locating myself in the network: I, an Einstein of sorts, had just discovered the theory of individual relativity.

While I was going through all these many transformations, I began to hear stories of women with breast cancer, friends of friends, who were wrestling with their own suffering. I was asked to talk with them on the telephone because they were all from out of state. We talked intimately, directly, with mutual respect for our suffering. They taught me something I had not known. They all had families who cared for them and wanted to help but did not know how. Their husbands, their children, their siblings, their parents were as frightened and shocked as the women were and could not find a way to deal with the deeper horror of the deadly threat. I had thought that I was unique because I had only a few relatives, and those spread far away. I was now learning from my conversations with these women that the confrontation with a deadly illness is a personal event that taxes the ordinary limits of human love. Love is not enough to help the sufferer. Deadly illness is a profound existential journey calling for a guide. Family and friends are indispensable to go through it. I could not have done it without my friends and the emotional support of my oncologist and nurse. Women my age frequently are alone because their children have their own families, are far away, have their own lives to tend to. And younger women usually have children who need them desperately and cannot postpone their urges until their mother is through with her ordeal. Their husbands have their own responsibilities and may be overwhelmed by pain. The extended family is in many cases geographically distant. Whatever the circumstance, any relative – husband, parent, older child, or sibling – who wants to help needs to become a friend capable of listening to the bewildered utterances of a very frightened human being. My friends have convinced me that this is the case, and I thank them for their tender faithfulness.

My life is now back to its ordinary routine. There are still subtle aspects of the act of being that require effort and attention. I feel an obscure fear of full engagement, of letting myself be taken over by the rhythm of what I am doing or partaking in. In short, I am afraid of living life as a dance with its own tune. Frequently, I discover I am searching for excuses not to be fully engaged. One day, while I was trying to understand my reticence, I recalled a traumatic moment of my childhood, when I was five years old. It was summertime and I had gone to the river's beach with my parents and siblings. My brother, sister, and I loved to build castles of sand. This time I had gone my own way to build a castle. I was totally absorbed in the task, full of fantasies about queens and kings. For that moment my life was taking place in the castle. My mother, who had lost sight of me for a long time, became worried and called me. I did not hear her voice until she was very close to me. Suddenly, she found me behind the rock where my castle was. In her panic, she shouted, "Why didn't you answer?" I was totally bewildered. I had not heard her. The transition from castles to reality had been too abrupt. It took me a few minutes to be able to enter the reality of my mother. I cried, in confusion, because I could not understand her anger. She tried to console me, but the episode left its mark.

The cancer had revived the pain of that unfortunate moment. I was afraid now of letting myself be fully involved in life only to feel – at the very moment of maximum absorption – the grip of cancer pulling me away from my engagement. This fear cut very deep. I have not found any remedy against it, except the courage to risk that such a thing might in fact happen. Thus, I came to see that the most courageous thing I could do was to let myself live fully, with passion, with involvement. I am trying to sustain the decision I feel is best for me: I want to be brave and to let myself love, create, laugh, cry, be engaged, accept with humility that I may be asked to surrender my life when I am having the greatest fun with it.

THE TENDER BUD

Made in the USA
Las Vegas, NV
24 June 2021